COOKING WITH CANNABIS

Delicious Recipes for Edibles and Everyday Favorites

LAURIE WOLF

MAKE YOUR MARRIAGE
DOWERIOUS! : Brooklyn
♡ Nichole & Brooklyn

QUARRY

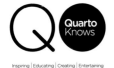

Brimming with creative inspiration, how-to projects, and useful information to enrich your everyday life, Quarto Knows is a favorite destination for those pursuing their interests and passions. Visit our site and dig deeper with our books into your area of interest: Quarto Creates, Quarto Cooks, Quarto Homes, Quarto Lives, Quarto Drives, Quarto Explores, Quarto Gifts, or Quarto Kids.

© 2016 Quarto Publishing Group USA Inc.
Text © 2016 Quarto Publishing Group USA Inc.
Photography © 2016 Bruce Wolf

First published in the United States of America in 2016 by
Quarry Books, an imprint of The Quarto Group,
100 Cummings Center, Suite 265-D, Beverly, MA 01915, USA.
T (978) 282-9590 F (978) 283-2742
QuartoKnows.com

Quarry Books Press titles are also available at discount for retail, wholesale, promotional, and bulk purchase. For details, contact the Special Sales Manager by email at specialsales@quarto.com or by mail at The Quarto Group, Attn: Special Sales Manager, 401 Second Avenue North, Suite 310, Minneapolis, MN 55401, USA.

10 9 8 7 6 5 4 3

ISBN: 978-1-63159-116-7

Digital edition published in 2016
eISBN: 978-1-63159-184-6

Library of Congress Cataloging-in-Publication Data is available

Design: Samantha J. Bednarek
Photography: Bruce Wolf

Printed in China

The information in this book is for educational purposes only. It is not intended to replace the advice of a physician or medical practitioner. Please see your health-care provider before beginning any new health program.

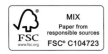

For Bruce and my kids. I love you.

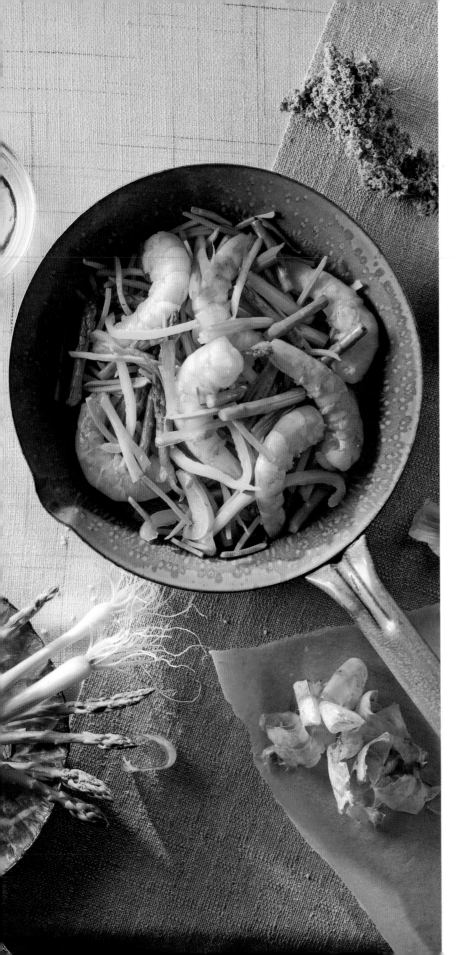

CONTENTS

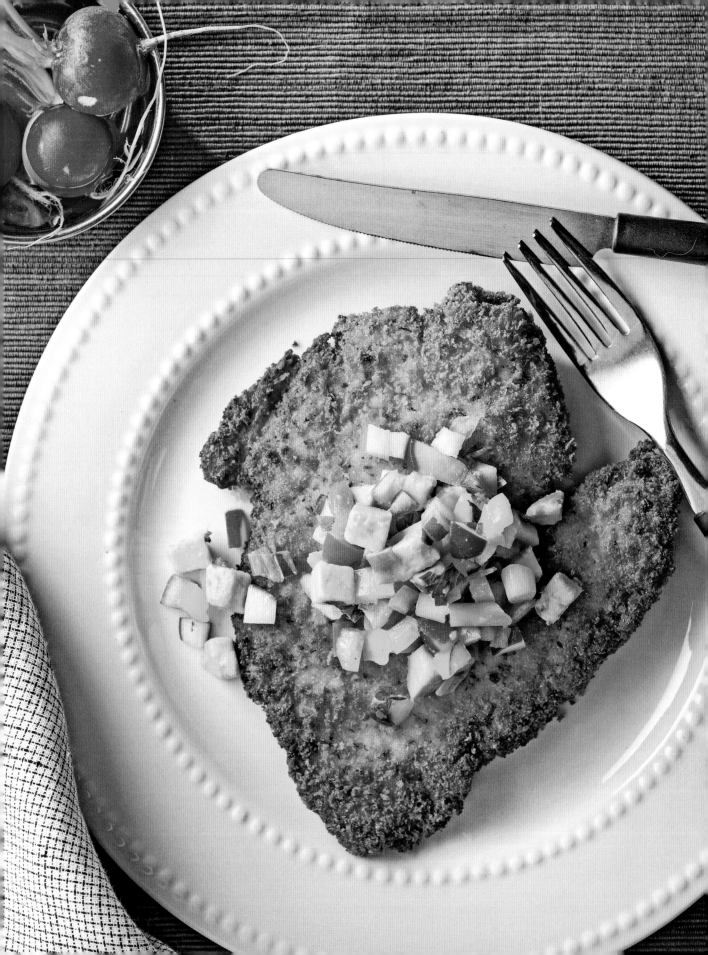

PREFACE

As I drive around Portland, Oregon, the city where I live, there are billboards advertising $79 prices for 1 ounce (28 g) of cannabis and others that promote cannabis concentrates. It's unbelievable. I never imagined that I would see this happen in my lifetime. I also never imagined that this was how I would make my living. I have an edibles company that sells products infused with marijuana. I'm a legal drug dealer, which still seems fairly hilarious.

For me, the most important benefit of the legalization of cannabis is that it allows people to use this plant to treat their health issues. Being able to control my epilepsy without using any pharmaceuticals has been life changing. For twenty years, I took medication that had extremely unpleasant and difficult to deal with side effects. My seizures stopped, though I continued to have pre-seizure auras monthly. But through using cannabis, for two years now I have been both seizure- and aura-free. That's right, not a hint; there are no side effects, and the amount of cannabis that I need for medicinal purposes does not make me uncomfortably high. That's pretty amazing.

I love that I have been able to help people with serious illnesses, including multiple sclerosis, fibromyalgia, and chronic nerve pain. Friends who could not tolerate pain medicine are getting serious relief from ingesting cannabis. I find it hard to imagine cannabis not being a better choice than Vicodin or hydrocodone. But that's me.

Having been in the cannabusiness for more than three years, I see that many folks just don't want to smoke. Ingesting cannabis, as long as you have the dosing down, is preferable and also a delightful way to medicate. As a cannabis chef, I love offering people infused edibles that are both nutritious and will also help them deal with health issues—as well as enjoying recreational cannabis in a safe manner.

Cannabis is here to stay. Whether you're going to use cannabis for health reasons or for fun, you need to understand the full picture. First, this is not your mother's cannabis! Second, there are strains that won't get you high, but that can help alleviate a headache or a stomach spasm. There's no reason why your cannabis experience should be anything but enjoyable, and I hope this book will serve as a trusted guide.

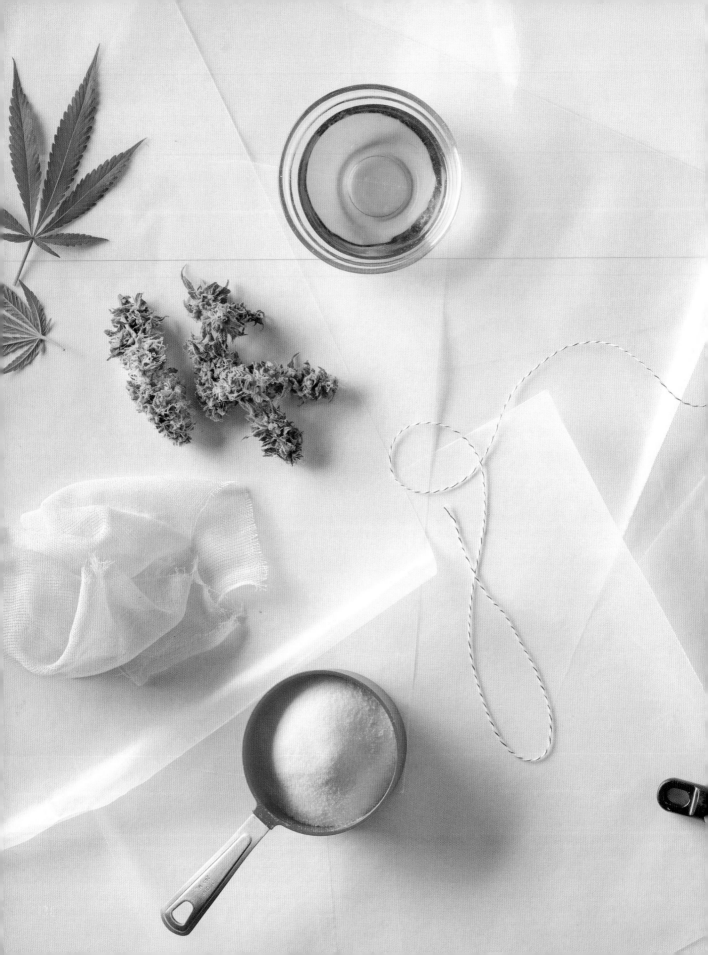

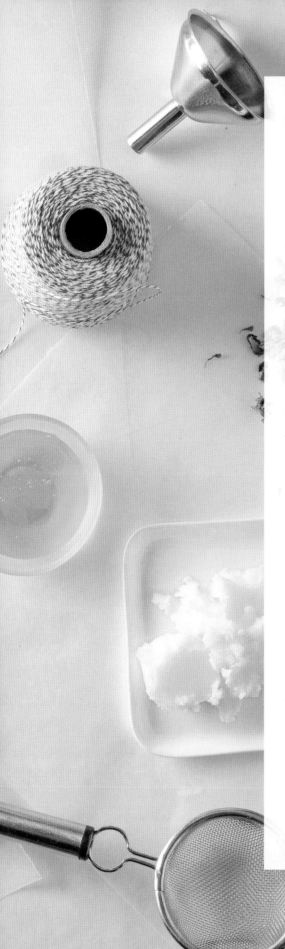

1

COOKING WITH CANNABIS: THE BASICS

Cooking with cannabis is akin to learning to cook with a new and distinctive herb. What I have found is that some foods work well with a hint of cannabis and some are better with no cannabis taste at all. Some foods, such as mushrooms and white chocolate, taste amazing with a good hit of cannabis. Infusing your cooking fat, whether it be butter or a cooking oil, is a simple process. As long as you follow the directions, you will have fabulous results. I "high"ly recommend it.

MARIJUANA: A CRASH COURSE

Cannabis was a prescribed drug in the United States until the early 1920s. Around that time, the Federal Bureau of Narcotics had it declared a hazard to society, and it was banned almost entirely. Things got even worse for the plant in the 1950s, when cannabis was declared a Schedule 1 drug, the highest category of drug classification in the United States, meaning the government does not recognize any accepted medical use for it. This situation continues today, and the federal government continues to consider marijuana to have high potential for abuse, with no legitimate medical or therapeutic use.

As states begin to decriminalize cannabis—at the time of this writing there are 23 states that have done so—there's hope that the federal government will change the status of cannabis. In states where cannabis is legal,

the federal government has declared that it would decline to enforce federal drug laws.

The compound in marijuana that has gotten the most attention is tetrahydrocannabinol, thankfully called THC for short. THC is what's responsible for the psychoactive or mind-altering effect of the plant. The THC cannabinoid, which is a chemical compound found in the cannabis plant resin, is responsible for pleasure, pain relief, time perception, and coordination. When THC enters the bloodstream, it activates neural receptors and causes the production of dopamine, the chemical in the brain that is responsible for feelings of euphoria. And who doesn't like feelings of euphoria?

More recently, the compound cannabidiol has been the buzz of the cannabis world. CBD for short, this cannabinoid has been found to be even more helpful than THC in treating pain, inflammation, and anxiety without the psychoactive effects of THC. Numerous medical studies are being published on a regular basis pointing to the many therapeutic effects of THC and, increasingly, CBD. Preliminary clinical studies suggest CBD may have therapeutic benefits in the treatment of chronic pain, arthritis, anxiety, cardiovascular disease, cancer, strokes, schizophrenia, PTSD, and diabetes. The high CBD strain of marijuana called Charlotte's Web was created by a group of brothers and popularized through its help with a young

THE MOST COMMON HEALTH ISSUES TREATED SUCCESSFULLY WITH CANNABIS

- AIDS/HIV
- Alzheimer's disease
- Anxiety
- Arthritis
- Asthma
- Cancer
- Chronic pain
- Crohn's disease
- Depression
- Epilepsy
- Glaucoma
- Insomnia
- Multiple sclerosis
- Nerve pain and fibromyalgia

PLAY IT SAFE.

Responsible cannabis use is as important as responsible alcohol use. Cannabis can be a powerful intoxicant if it's used incorrectly, so it's absolutely essential that you follow—no, memorize—these safety tips before you try any of the recipes in this book.

- **Cannabis isn't kid-friendly.** Cannabis products should never be given to children unless specifically recommended by a medical doctor. Be sure to keep your cannabis and cannabis-infused products safely away from kids.

- **Start with—and consider sticking with— a very small dose.** As with food in general, so with cannabis: You can always add more spice if you need to, but you can't take it out once you've added it, so proceed with care. And if you do use too much cannabis extract in your food, stay put. Ask for help if you need it, and whatever you do, don't make any plans to drive.

- **Pay attention to your body's unique reactions.** Each person's tolerance for cannabis is different, and can be influenced by factors such as your lifestyle, your psychological or emotional state, and any medications you might be taking. That's why you need to be mindful of your individual reactions to cannabis. Know your personal limits, and don't exceed them: If you start to feel unwell, stop consuming cannabis immediately.

- **Cannabis impairs decision-making and motor skills.** That's why it's important to consume cannabis in a safe place—in your own home, for instance, or in the company of someone you trust.

- **Side effects may take a while to wear off.** It's important to be aware that some side effects of consuming cannabis can last for up to 24 hours after ingestion. Always plan your schedule accordingly. Common side effects include dizziness, tiredness, and nausea.

- **Consult your doctor before use.** As with any type of herbal medicine, you should always consult your doctor before you attempt any non–FDA approved practices.

girl's seemingly impossible fight against a rare form of epilepsy. This strain has allowed her, and many like her, to lead a normal life. The results have been outstanding, and growers are working to develop more strains of marijuana that are high in CBD. That being said, there's still a considerable amount of research needed to validate the stories of patients like this little girl.

Effects of ingesting the plant will vary depending on the strain used; in addition, individual people may have different experiences from ingesting the same strain. While inhaling will affect you nearly immediately, ingesting takes 30 minutes to 3 hours to reach the full effect. The high from ingesting also lasts for a much longer time and has a stronger, more sedative effect than the high from inhaling. As with most things, individuals are affected in different ways by different things, so always start small.

INDICAS, SATIVAS, AND HYBRIDS

Sativa and indica are the two major subspecies of the cannabis plant. When bred together, the results are called hybrids. In dispensaries, you'll generally find all three. Each strain (a genetic variant or subtype) affects the mind and body differently.

Indica strains typically produce a high that manifests itself in a physical way, while the sativa strains tend to produce a high that's more cerebral. The differences between the strains can be pretty subtle, but there are strains that are clearly uplifting (sativas) or sedating (indicas).

Indica strains are recommended for pain relief as well as for help with anxiety and stress reduction. If you're looking for a relaxing night on the couch or you want a good night's sleep, indicas are the way to go. Indica strains tend to have a higher CBD percentage and a stronger all-around analgesic effect.

Sativa strains are best suited for daytime use, as the effects are associated with increased energy, euphoria, creativity, and focus. But with these effects can sometimes come anxiety and paranoia. For some people, sativas help fight depression. If you're looking for an intense and stimulating cerebral experience, sativas are the way to go. And you can certainly enjoy the benefits of a sativa without ending up with an intense reaction.

With all the crossbreeding and hybridizations going on out there, the lines have gotten very blurred between indicas and sativas. The emerging thought is that the varying effects can be attributed to the terpene profile of the plant. Terpenes are the organic compounds—oils, actually—in cannabis and other plants that determine their smell. There are over 100 terpenes found in the cannabis plant, and they're thought to be able to increase the potency of THC and other cannabinoids. Some of the most common terpenes, for example, are pinene, myrcene, limonene, and linalool. In addition to affecting the smell and taste of the cannabis, these compounds also impact the physical and psychological effects.

Another element responsible for the varying effects of cannabis is the cannabinoid ratio; that is, the ratio of THC to CBD in a particular strain.

When purchasing cannabis, try to find a dispensary where the budtenders are knowledgeable and are clearly listening when you explain what you're looking for. If you're a patient who wants only the medicinal benefits of cannabis without feeling a difference mentally, that should be possible. More and more strains are becoming available that have a higher CBD percentage than THC.

Much more research is needed to test these theories. Until then, talk to your budtenders, read reviews online, and keep a journal of your experiences with different strains.

DOSING: LESS IS MORE

Ingesting too much cannabis is extremely unpleasant. It's not harmful, but just a guaranteed miserable time. You may experience dizziness, nausea, disorientation, and a "please let this pass" kind of feeling. Never eat more than is recommended in the recipe serving sizes. Know what you're putting into your body and always remember: Less is more.

Every individual has a different tolerance, so there are no hard and fast rules for dosing. To figure out what your own personal tolerance is, perform a test by trying a very small amount of an infused base product, like the Canna-Oil (page 18) or Canna-Butter (page 16). I suggest ¼ teaspoon to start. Wait for 3 hours to get the full effect. It doesn't usually take that long, but it can take anywhere from 30 minutes to 3 hours, so be patient. You can then try another test if necessary or desired using a slightly greater amount of the infused base product. Once you know your dosing parameters through this experimentation, you will be able to avoid going overboard. If you make an infusion that you feel is too strong, dilute it with plain butter or oil, depending on your infusion.

Although medical patients may require very high doses to find relief, recreational users are often quite happy with 5 mg of THC. Personally, I am good with a 10 mg THC dose. When purchasing from dispensaries, information on dosing for the different strains will be available. Although it may not make sense, sometimes a lower dose makes for a better time. If you get too out of it, you miss all the fun.

WHAT TO DO WHEN YOU OVERDO IT

- Take a dose of ibuprofen. It will take about 30 minutes to kick in, but it has been shown to lessen the effects of THC.

- Drink water. It will make you feel better and help your body process the excess THC.

- Citrus is thought to help relieve symptoms of being too high, particularly freshly squeezed lemon juice.

- Keep a high CBD strain in your house. CBD is thought to lessen the effects of THC. Smoking or vaping a couple of hits can provide some quick relief.

- Try to sleep. Get yourself as comfortable as you can and tuck yourself into bed. Keep your eyes closed and focus on rhythmic breathing.

- Marijuana is nonfatal and there is no risk of an overdose. Remember that this unpleasant feeling will wear off—but probably not as quickly as you would like!

STORING AND FREEZING CANNABIS AND EDIBLES

Store cannabis in glass jars with tight-fitting lids. Keep the jars in a cool, dark place. I have kept jars of cannabis this way for more than a year without any loss of potency. You want to keep your cannabis in a spot that has a consistent amount of light and a consistent temperature; fluctuations of both can have a negative effect on the plant. If you can vacuum-seal the jars, that would be ideal. Dark-colored glass jars add an extra layer of protection against light. Remember to keep your strains labeled and in their own containers, ensuring that you will keep their taste, smell, and potency from changing.

The greatest enemies when storing cannabis are excessive heat and sunlight. When exposed to direct sunlight or high temperatures, the cannabinoids and terpenes will degrade. And warm air is a carrier of both mold and mildew. Additionally, very low temperatures can have an adverse effect on cannabis. Forget the freezer because it can freeze the trichomes (the little hair-like filaments) and they will break off, lowering the potency. The refrigerator is also not a good place to store cannabis as the humidity can lead to the growth of mold and mildew. Be sure that your cannabis is dry when you are placing it in jars for storage or else you will have another opportunity for mold and mildew growth.

When storing edibles made with Canna-Butter or Canna-Oil, follow the same guidelines that would be appropriate for any non-infused food. Anything that can be frozen when made without cannabis can still go in the freezer with cannabis. I like to freeze all baked products, whether sweets like cookies or savories like casseroles, double wrapped. First I wrap them in parchment paper and then in aluminum foil or plastic wrap. If the product is not fragile, I use plastic food-storage bags that I can vacuum-seal. Let foods come to room temperature before eating (if you aren't reheating them), as they will taste better. I have included more specific storage information with individual recipes.

DECARBOXYLATION

In order to derive the greatest potency from the cannabis plant when making edibles, it's best to always decarboxylate the cannabis before infusing. Decarboxylation is the process of heating the marijuana to activate both the THC and the CBD in the plant. This heating happens naturally when you are smoking or vaping the plant, but when ingesting marijuana, you should first decarb it.

While we have enjoyed excellent results without first decarbing, our lab tests indicate that there is a small but worthwhile increase in potency when the plant is first decarbed. Decarbing versus not decarbing does not seem to affect the shelf life of either the cannabis or the finished food made with it. If you have the time, I suggest you take this extra step. It's a very simple procedure; follow these instructions using any amount of cannabis (buds or trim):

1. Preheat the oven to 240°F (115°C, or gas mark ½). Break apart any large buds with your hands and spread the cannabis on a rimmed baking sheet (fig. 1).
2. Bake for 45 minutes. The cannabis should become lightly browned and at this point will be decarboxylated (fig. 2).

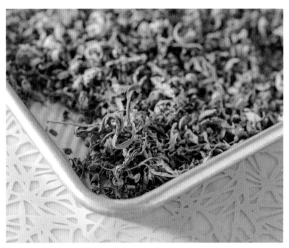

1. Spread the cannabis on a rimmed baking sheet.

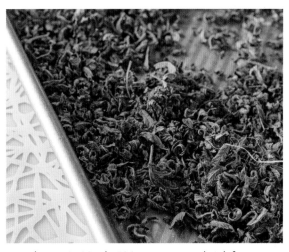

2. Bake at 240°F (115°C, or gas mark ½) for 45 minutes.

CHEF'S NOTE

When you decarboxylate at a low temperature, as here, you are preserving the most terpenes, which are the oils in the cannabis that influence its flavor profile and provide some of the health benefits.

CANNA-BUTTER

Follow these directions and you'll make the best Canna-Butter your ingredients will allow. Bear in mind that the stronger the strain, the stronger the butter, so plan accordingly. To grind the cannabis, you may use a blender or food processor or do it by hand.

1 **quart (946 ml) water**

1 **pound (455 g) butter**

1 **ounce (28 g) cannabis, decarboxylated (page 15) and finely ground**

1. In a medium saucepan, bring the water to a boil. You can vary the amount of water if you like; just be sure to use enough so the cannabis is always floating 1½ to 2 inches (4 to 5 cm) from the bottom of the pan. Place the butter in the saucepan (fig. 1).

2. Once the butter has melted completely, add the cannabis (fig. 2).

3. Reduce the heat to very low to simmer. Cook for about 3 hours. It's done when the surface of the mixture turns from really watery to glossy and thick (fig. 3).

4. While the Canna-Butter is cooking, set up a bowl to hold the finished product. There are a couple of ways to strain the mixture. I like to wrap a double layer of cheesecloth around a large heatproof bowl with kitchen twine, making sure the cheesecloth is taut across the top of the bowl. Carefully strain the Canna-Butter into the bowl, working slowly to avoid spills (fig. 4).

5. When the saucepan is empty, carefully untie the twine, pick up the cheesecloth on all four sides, and squeeze out all of the remaining liquid (fig. 5).

6. Allow to cool at room temperature for about 1 hour. Refrigerate until the butter has solidified and separated from the water (fig. 6).

7. Place a sheet of parchment paper on your work surface. Run a knife around the edge of the Canna-Butter and lift it off the water (fig. 7). Place the Canna-Butter upside down on the parchment paper and lightly scrape off any remaining cooking water (fig. 8). Use the parchment paper to shape and roll the Canna-Butter into a cylinder. Store in an airtight container in the refrigerator for up to 1 month or in the freezer for up to 6 months.

Yield: Makes 1 pound (455 g)

CHEF'S NOTE The ratio for this recipe is 1 pound (455 g) of butter to every 1 ounce (28 g) of marijuana. That means that if you're using ½ ounce (15 g) of cannabis, you'll need about ½ pound (225 g) of butter.

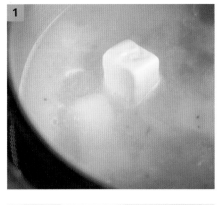

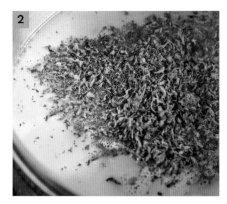

1. Melt the butter in boiling water.

2. Stir in the cannabis.

3. Cook over very low heat.

4. Carefully strain through cheesecloth.

5. Squeeze to remove the remaining liquid.

6. Let cool and then refrigerate until solidified.

7. Run a knife around the edge to release from the bowl.

8. Place upside down on parchment paper and remove any remaining liquid.

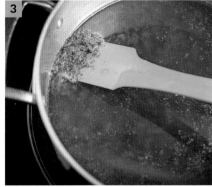

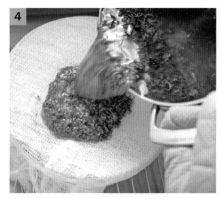

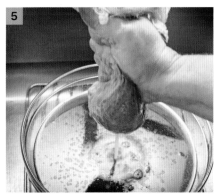

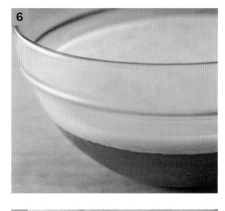

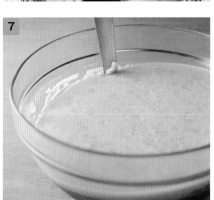

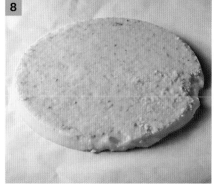

CANNA-OIL

The steps to infusing oil are the same regardless of the type of oil used. You can even make a blend of oils if you like. My favorite is coconut oil: It infuses beautifully and can even be used as a topical remedy. In addition to being used in many recipes in this book, you can also use Canna-Oil to make mayonnaise and vinaigrette (see Cannabis Condiments, page 20). If a recipe does not specify Canna-Oil made with a particular type of oil, use whatever Canna-Oil you like or have on hand.

2 **cups (475 ml) canola, (475 ml) olive, or (455 g) coconut oil**

1 **ounce (28 g) cannabis, decarboxylated (page 15) and finely ground**

1. In a medium saucepan, heat the oil over medium-low heat. Add the cannabis (fig. 1).

2. Simmer gently for 3 hours. Do not allow the oil to come to a boil. Cooking at a very low simmer, with occasional bubbles, is the desired method. You can tell the oil is done when the top of the mixture turns from watery to glossy and thick (fig. 2).

3. Carefully pour the oil and cannabis into your prepared bowl. There are a couple of ways to do the straining. I like to use a deep heatproof glass bowl with a fine-mesh strainer lined with cheesecloth (fig. 3). You can also tie a double layer of cheesecloth around a large heatproof bowl with kitchen twine, making it taut across the top.

4. When the saucepan is empty, carefully undo the twine, pick up the cheesecloth from all four sides, and squeeze out all of the remaining oil (fig. 4).

5. Allow the Canna-Oil to cool at room temperature for about 1 hour (fig. 5). Pour into a glass jar with a lid and store in the refrigerator for up to 6 months.

Yield: Makes 2 cups (475 ml)

CHEF'S NOTE

The technique of oil infusion varies from the butter procedure because the process for oil doesn't involve water. Water is used in the butter infusion to help prevent the milk solids from burning. Also, since butter becomes solid in the refrigerator, it's easy to remove the butter from the water.

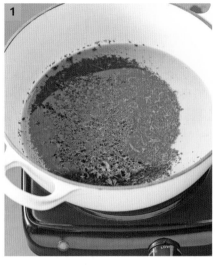

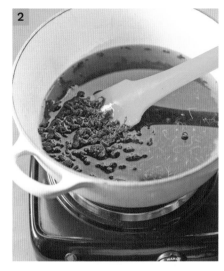

1. Heat the oil and then add the cannabis.

2. Simmer gently for 3 hours.

3. Strain through cheesecloth. Work carefully to avoid spills.

4. Squeeze to remove the remaining oil.

5. Let cool. Pour into a glass jar with a lid and store in the refrigerator.

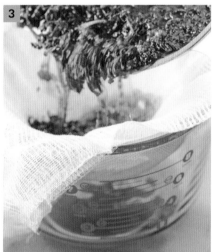

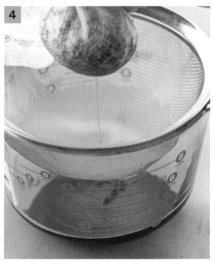

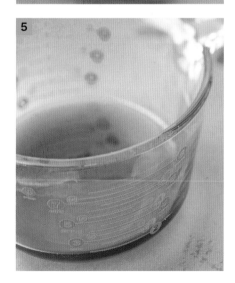

CANNABIS CONDIMENTS

When using infused condiments, such as this mayonnaise and vinaigrette, it's best to omit any other cannabis from the recipe. The recipes in this book were created to give you a dose that's reasonable without being overpowering. If you're a medical patient and know what your dose is, you may decide to use the infused condiment along with the recipe, but this approach is only for folks who can handle higher doses. Whether you're working with your doctor or with a budtender, remember that less is more unless you truly know how much cannabis you can ingest.

Canna-Mayonnaise

3   large egg yolks

2   teaspoons fresh lemon juice

1   teaspoon Dijon mustard

½   cup (120 ml) Canna-Oil (page 18)

½   cup (120 ml) olive oil

     Pinch of salt

1. In the bowl of a food processor, combine the egg yolks, lemon juice, and Dijon mustard. Process to combine.
2. With the machine running, drizzle in the oils. Add the salt. The mixture will get thick. If necessary, add a drop or two of water to achieve the desired consistency. Store in an airtight container in the refrigerator for up to 1 week.

Yield: 2 cups (450 g)

Canna-Vinaigrette

6   tablespoons (90 ml) balsamic vinegar

1   tablespoon (15 g) Dijon mustard

1   clove of garlic, minced

½   cup (120 ml) Canna-Oil (page 18)

½   cup (120 ml) olive oil

     Salt and black pepper

In a medium bowl, combine the balsamic vinegar, Dijon mustard, and garlic. Drizzle in the oils in a slow stream, whisking constantly. Season with salt and black pepper to taste. Store in an airtight container in the refrigerator for up to 3 months.

Yield: 1½ cups (355 ml)

SNACK ATTACKS:
10 EASY-TO-MAKE SNACKS WHEN YOU'RE UNDER THE INFLUENCE

For those occasions when the munchies kick in and you're not in the mood to cook, here's a list of ten of the most satisfying, un-infused snacks with three ingredients or fewer.

1. Ricotta cheese, chocolate chips, and vanilla, mixed together in a bowl: It's easy and tasty, like a cannoli filling without the shell!

2. Cinnamon toast: This childhood snack is too good to be forgotten. You just need bread, butter, sugar or honey, and cinnamon. Oh yeah, and a toaster!

3. Banana slices drizzled with coconut cream and sprinkled with brown sugar: Coconut cream is not the very sweet piña colada coconut product. It's thick and mild and you will love it with brown sugar. Vegans, go with agave nectar.

4. Berries, whipped Greek yogurt, and honey: If you can whip the yogurt, it will be fluffy and awesome. If you can't, it will just be awesome!

5. Radishes with butter and salt: The better the butter, the more delish it will be. Sea salt is best.

6. Fried cheese: You just need a nonstick skillet and the cheese of your choice. I like cheddar. This snack is like the little gooey bits that cook and brown in the pan after they falls out of your grilled cheese sandwich.

7. Avocado drizzled with olive oil, balsamic vinegar, and salt and black pepper: Just halve the avocado, remove the pit, sprinkle on the toppings, and eat with a spoon.

8. Flour tortillas baked with olive oil and coarse salt: Brush tortilla wedges with oil and sprinkle with salt. Place on a baking sheet and cook in a 300°F (150°C, or gas mark 2) oven until golden brown, turning once. Use your mitts to turn them. Allow to cool. Use your mitts. Don't forget.

9. Corn kernels with mayo and chili powder: Briefly sauté the corn, let cool, and toss with a bit of mayo, some chili powder, and salt. It's like Mexican corn, but off the cob.

10. Cottage cheese and honey on whole-grain bread: Toasting the bread is optional.

SIMPLE CANNA-SYRUP

Simple syrup is a must if you love a good cocktail, and what a lovely infusion this simple syrup turned out to be. This process produces a syrup that's less psychoactive than butter or oil. It's a fabulous way to make some wonderful canna-cocktails, and it's also great for sweetening coffee, tea, smoothies, granitas, and more. You can make any amount of syrup; just use equal parts water and sugar.

3 **cups (700 ml) filtered water**

3 **cups (600 g) granulated sugar**

½ **ounce (15 g) cannabis, decarboxylated (page 15) and finely chopped**

3 **tablespoons (45 ml) vegetable glycerin**

1. In a large saucepan, bring the water to a boil (fig. 1). Add the sugar and stir until dissolved (fig. 2).

2. Add the cannabis, cover, and reduce the heat to a simmer. Simmer for 30 minutes (fig. 3).

3. Reduce the heat to low, stir in the glycerin, and simmer for 10 minutes (fig. 4). Remove from the heat and let cool for 20 minutes.

4. Place a layer of cheesecloth or a fine-mesh strainer over a heatproof bowl or jar and carefully pour the syrup into the bowl, straining out the cannabis (fig. 5). Allow the syrup to cool to room temperature.

5. Place the syrup into a jar or other container with a tight-fitting lid. Store in the refrigerator for up to 3 months (fig. 6).

Yield: 4 cups (946 ml)

CHEF'S NOTE The cannabis infuses the sugar-water mixture with the help of the glycerin, which aids the emulsification process.

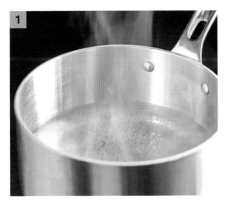

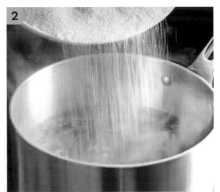

1. Bring the water to a boil.

2. Add the sugar. Stir to dissolve.

3. Add the cannabis. Reduce the heat and simmer for 30 minutes.

4. Add the glycerin and simmer for 10 minutes.

5. Remove from the heat, let cool slightly, and then strain.

6. Cool to room temperature. Cover and refrigerate.

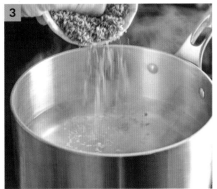

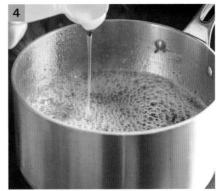

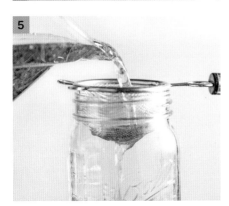

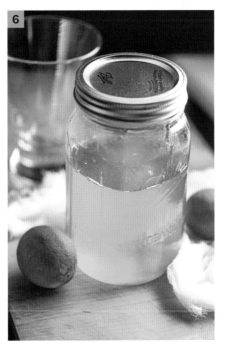

CANNA-CREAM

This ratio of ingredients makes a strong cannabis cream. Feel free to lessen the potency by adding additional heavy cream or using less cannabis. It's great for using in hot drinks and for whipping and topping desserts.

2 cups (475 ml) heavy cream

½ ounce (15 g) cannabis, decarboxylated (page 15) and finely chopped

1. In a double boiler over medium heat or in a medium bowl set on top of a saucepan partially filled with water, heat the cream until it just starts to bubble. Add the cannabis to the hot cream (fig. 1).

2. Use a spatula to fold the cannabis into the cream (fig. 2) and then whisk to combine thoroughly. Lower the heat and simmer very gently for 1 hour (fig. 3).

3. Carefully pour the mixture through a fine-mesh strainer lined with cheesecloth into a bowl (fig. 4). Let cool at room temperature for 20 minutes.

4. Cover and refrigerate for about 1 week (fig. 5).

Yield: Makes 2 cups (475 ml)

CHEF'S NOTE

The green cream makes quite a statement. The test results from our lab, Chem History, show that the potency of the infused cream is less than, but close to, the strength of Canna-Butter (page 16) and Canna-Oil (page 18). This makes sense because the THC likes to have a fat to cling to during the infusing process.

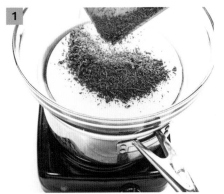

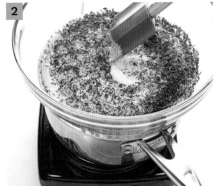

1. Heat the cream and then add the cannabis.

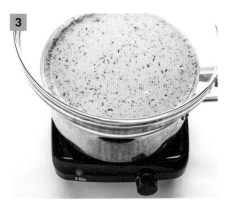

2. Fold in the cannabis and then whisk to combine.

3. Gently simmer for 1 hour.

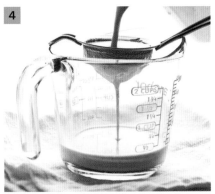

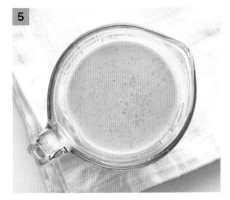

4. Strain through a cheesecloth-lined strainer.

5. Cover and refrigerate. Use within 1 week.

CANNA-FLOUR

Not a method I use often, Canna-Flour involves baking with the actual plant. This means more of that cannabis flavor than you would get from the other infusions. But it also means fewer steps!

1 ounce (28 g) cannabis, decarboxylated (page 15)

1. Place the cannabis in the bowl of your food processor or in a clean coffee grinder (fig. 1). Process to a very fine flour-like powder (fig. 2). Stored in an airtight container, it will keep for many months (fig. 3).

2. To use, replace up to one-quarter of the amount of flour called for in a recipe with cannabis flour (fig. 4). Sift together the prepared cannabis flour with the other flour for even distribution.

Yield: Makes 1 cup (125 g)

CHEF'S NOTE For the sake of flavor and consistency in the finished product, try to stay at or below the one-quarter substitution rule. When baking with Canna-Flour, keep the oven at 340°F (170°C, or gas mark 3) or below. For recipes that call for 350°F (180°C, or gas mark 4), just lower the oven temperature to 340°F (170°C, or gas mark 3) and cook for a few minutes longer. Ramp up the seasonings a bit and there should be no harsh taste of cannabis.

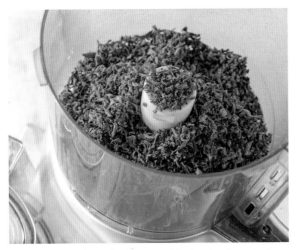

1. Place the decarbed cannabis in the bowl of a food processor.

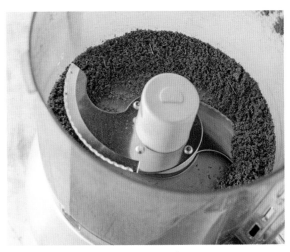

2. Process to a very fine powder.

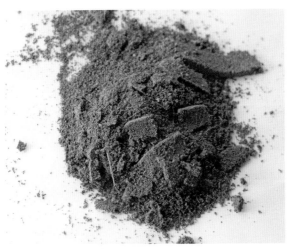

3. Once processed, store in an airtight container until needed.

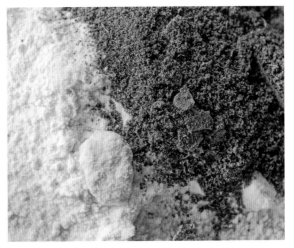

4. Sift together the Canna-Flour and other flour before using.

CANNA-HONEY

I had an interesting experience with this honey infusion. Testing indicated that very little of the THC was absorbed into the honey, rendering it only very mildly psychotropic. My business partner and I tested the honey three times, always getting the same results. From my personal experience, the infused honey seems to be physically relaxing, and 1 tablespoon (20 g) is potent enough to be calming and to help with sleep.

½ **ounce (15 g) cannabis, decarboxylated (page 15) and finely chopped**

4 **cups (1.3 kg) honey**

1. Place the cannabis in a cheesecloth bag or pouch tied with kitchen twine (fig. 1).
2. In a medium saucepan over medium heat, bring the honey to a simmer (fig. 2). Add the cheesecloth with the cannabis to the honey and simmer gently over low heat for 2 to 3 hours (fig. 3).
3. Remove the cheesecloth and squeeze to extract all the honey (be careful, as it will be very hot). Let cool at room temperature. Store indefinitely in a covered jar in the refrigerator.

Yield: Makes 4 cups (1.3 kg)

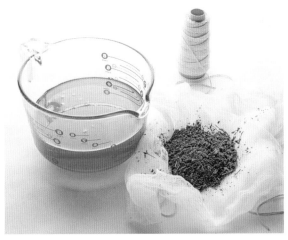

1. Place the cannabis in a cheesecloth pouch.

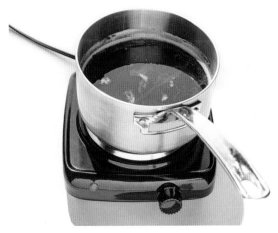

2. Bring the honey to a simmer.

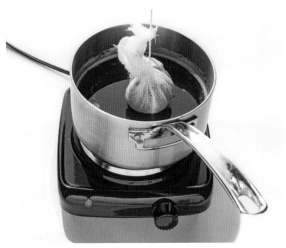

3. Place the pouch in the honey and simmer gently for 2 to 3 hours.

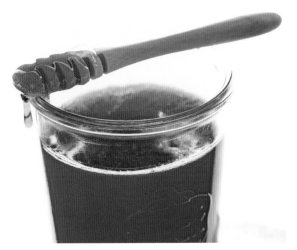

4. Let cool and refrigerate to store.

CANNA-HERB BLENDS

If you're looking for an easy way to get a mild high, you can sprinkle your food with a Canna-Herb Blend. Even a very strong strain won't be too much if you use just a little. An herb blend is also a nice way to start enjoying the flavor of cannabis if you don't already.

I discovered the potential of seasoning with cannabis by accident, when some of my decarboxylated weed ended up on my marinated skirt steak. Fortunately, when it kicked in I was the only one eating and was home for the night! I make a lot of this mix when my garden is at its peak. I've also added the dried herb blend to olive oil or melted butter—then it's a quick drizzle over food rather than a sprinkle.

¼ **ounce (7 g) cannabis**

¼ **ounce (7 g) fresh lemon thyme leaves**

¼ **ounce (7 g) fresh oregano leaves**

1. Preheat the oven to 200°F (93°C, or gas mark ¼). Place the cannabis and the herbs on a rimmed baking sheet (fig. 1).

2. Bake for 60 minutes until the herbs have dried out and turned brown (fig. 2). Allow to cool completely.

3. Place in the bowl of a food processor and pulse until coarsely chopped (fig. 3).

4. When stored in a jar with a tight-fitting lid and out of direct sunlight (fig. 4), this blend seems to keep indefinitely, though the herbs will lose their fragrance over time.

CHEF'S NOTE

The options for a Canna-Herb Blend are many. I've also had great success using a combination of dill and parsley, as well as thyme and rosemary.

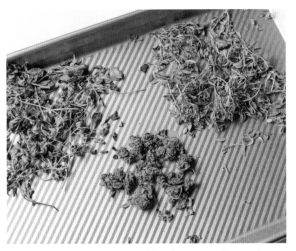

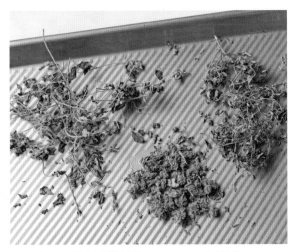

1. Place the cannabis and herbs on a rimmed baking sheet.

2. Bake at 200°F (90°C, or gas mark ¼) for 60 minutes.

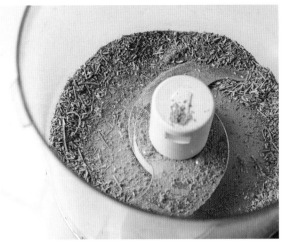

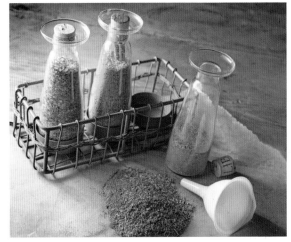

3. In a food processor, pulse until coarsely ground.

4. Store in a tightly closed jar away from direct sunlight.

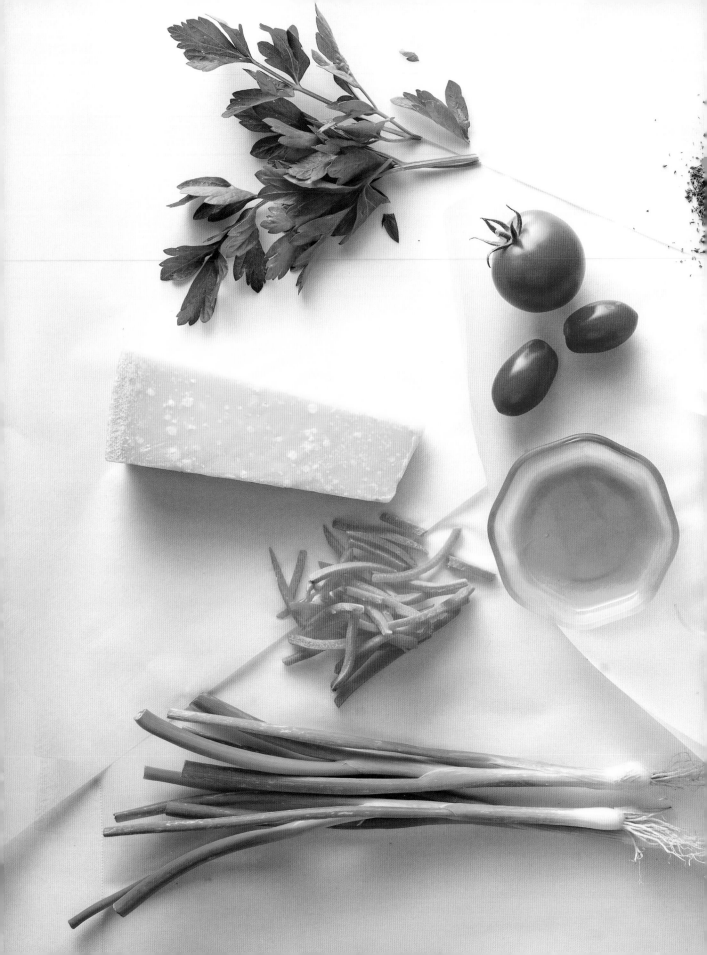

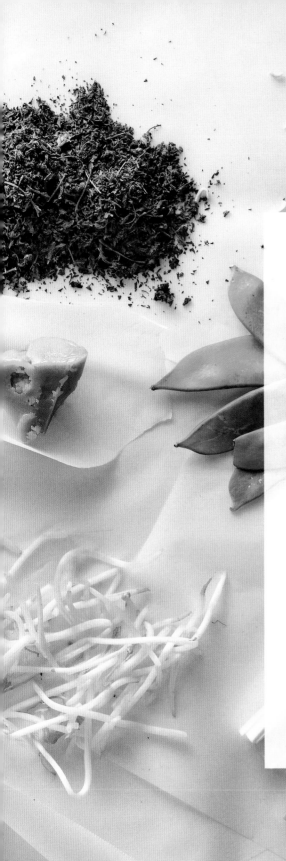

2

RECIPES FOR ONE

Eating alone at home has a lot going for it. There's no pressure to entertain anyone, you can make whatever it is that you're in the mood to eat, and you don't have to share. Whether you watch TV, read a book, or listen to music while you eat, it's your decision. Enjoy it as a time to reflect, to rejoice—and maybe even to eat with your fingers!

SIMPLE BUTTERNUT SQUASH SOUP

• **Gluten-free**

This simple-to-make soup is sure to warm you on cold winter nights. If you have the time, roast the squash instead of boiling it. Doing so adds a wonderful level of complexity. The avocado garnish is terrific, but so are fried sage leaves, a dollop of crème fraîche, or a simple sprinkling of smoked paprika.

1 teaspoon Canna-Butter (page 16)

1 teaspoon unsalted butter

¼ cup (40 g) chopped yellow onion

2 tablespoons (16 g) peeled and chopped carrot

1½ cups (210 g) peeled, seeded, and chopped butternut squash (may be substituted with cubed frozen squash)

¾ cup (175 ml) low-sodium gluten-free chicken broth

5 smoked almonds, coarsely chopped

Salt and black pepper

Chunks of avocado tossed with lemon juice, for garnish

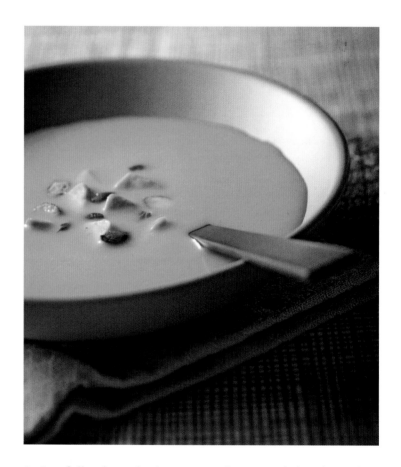

1. Place both butters in a small saucepan over medium-low heat. Add the onion and carrot and sauté until the onion is translucent, about 6 to 7 minutes.

2. Add the squash and chicken broth and simmer until the squash is tender, about 20 minutes.

3. Carefully place the hot soup mixture and the almonds in a blender and puree until smooth. Season with salt and black pepper to taste.

4. Pour the soup into a bowl and top with the avocado chunks.

Yield: Serves 1

SHRIMP AND ASPARAGUS STIR-FRY

Asparagus and shrimp are a great flavor combination. This dish is quick and easy to pull together. All you need is a bowl of rice and you're in business. It might be considered cheating, but I often just heat up the rice from some leftover takeout when I make this dish.

- 2 tablespoons (32 ml) hoisin sauce
- 2 teaspoons soy sauce
- 1 teaspoon Canna-Oil (page 18)
- 2 tablespoons (28 ml) canola oil
- 5 stalks of asparagus, woody stems removed and cut into pieces
- ¼ cup (28 g) shredded carrots
- ½ of a yellow bell pepper, sliced
- 8 medium shrimp, peeled, tails removed
- 2 scallions, sliced
- ½ teaspoon minced fresh ginger
- 1 clove of garlic, peeled and minced
- 1 teaspoon sesame seeds

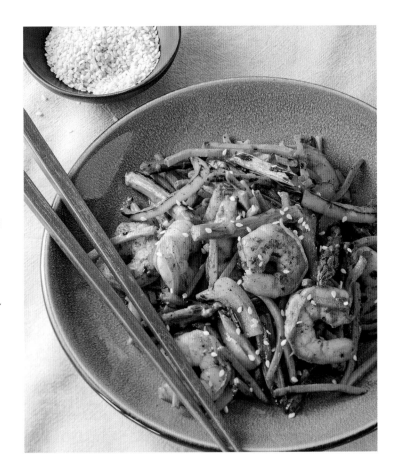

1. In a small bowl, combine the hoisin and soy sauces with the Canna-Oil and set aside.

2. In a large sauté pan, heat the canola oil over medium-high heat. Add the asparagus, carrots, and bell pepper and stir quickly for 4 to 5 minutes. Add the shrimp and cook until they turn pink and are firm to the touch, about 3 to 4 minutes. Stir in the scallions, ginger, and garlic.

3. Add the sauce to the pan and toss to evenly distribute the ingredients. Sprinkle with the sesame seeds and enjoy.

Yield: Serves 1

CHEF'S NOTE You can substitute green beans for the asparagus and tofu or chicken for the shrimp.

SUPER RAMEN

Ramen noodles are amazing. I was introduced to them by my son Nick, when he was in college. Clearly a simple package of ramen needs no directions, but I have ramped up the ingredients and added a little canna-love. When you mix the Canna-Oil with sesame oil, a totally awesome flavor combination emerges. Check your fridge: There is bound to be something in there to add to your soup. For a heartier meal, add some cooked chicken, shrimp, or tofu.

1   package (3½ ounces, or 100 g) ramen noodles

2   cups (475 ml) water or chicken or vegetable broth

¼   cup (9 g) packed watercress

1   scallion, sliced

6   sugar snap peas, halved

¼   cup (28 g) shredded carrots

1   large soft-boiled egg, peeled and halved

¼   cup (26 g) sprouts of your choice

    Fresh cilantro leaves, for garnish

2   teaspoons toasted sesame oil

1   teaspoon Canna-Oil (page 18)

1. Open the package of ramen and remove the flavor packet. Add the water or broth to a medium saucepan and bring to a boil.

2. Add the watercress, scallion, and noodles to the pot and simmer for 3 to 4 minutes. Add the peas and carrots along with the flavor packet from your package of ramen and cook for 1 minute.

3. Pour the soup into a bowl, add the egg, sprouts, cilantro, and both oils and serve.

Yield: Serves 1

CHEF'S NOTE I like to get the packages of ramen noodles that don't have MSG in the ingredients. MSG makes me feel weird, and it's pretty simple to avoid it. If you feel the same way but can't find ramen noodles without it, don't use the flavor packet. Instead, add some tamari sauce along with the peas and carrots and use chicken or vegetable broth instead of water.

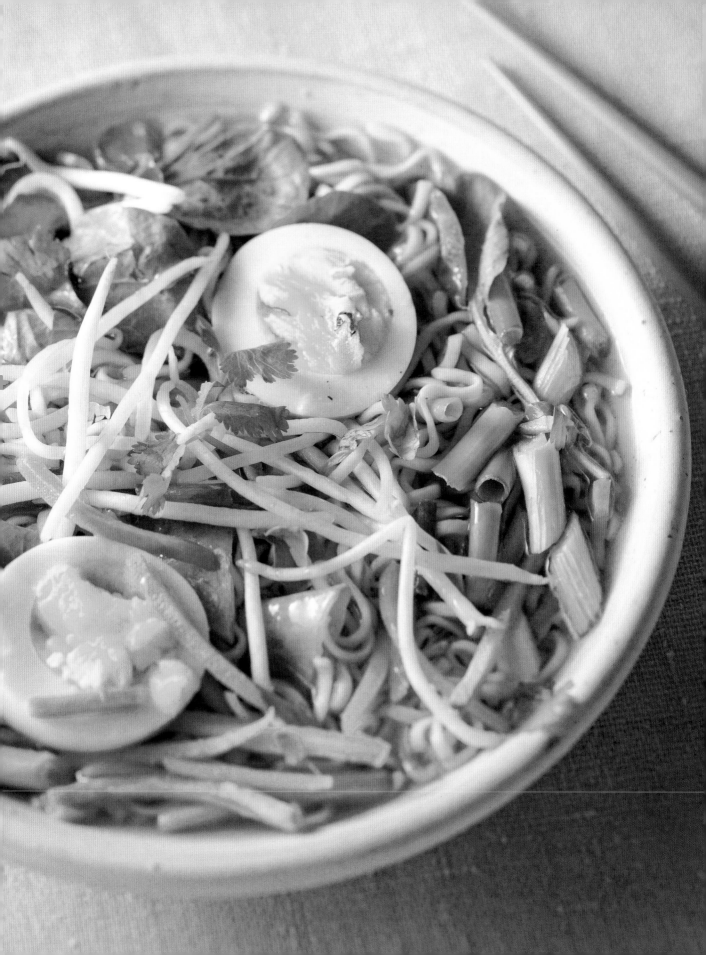

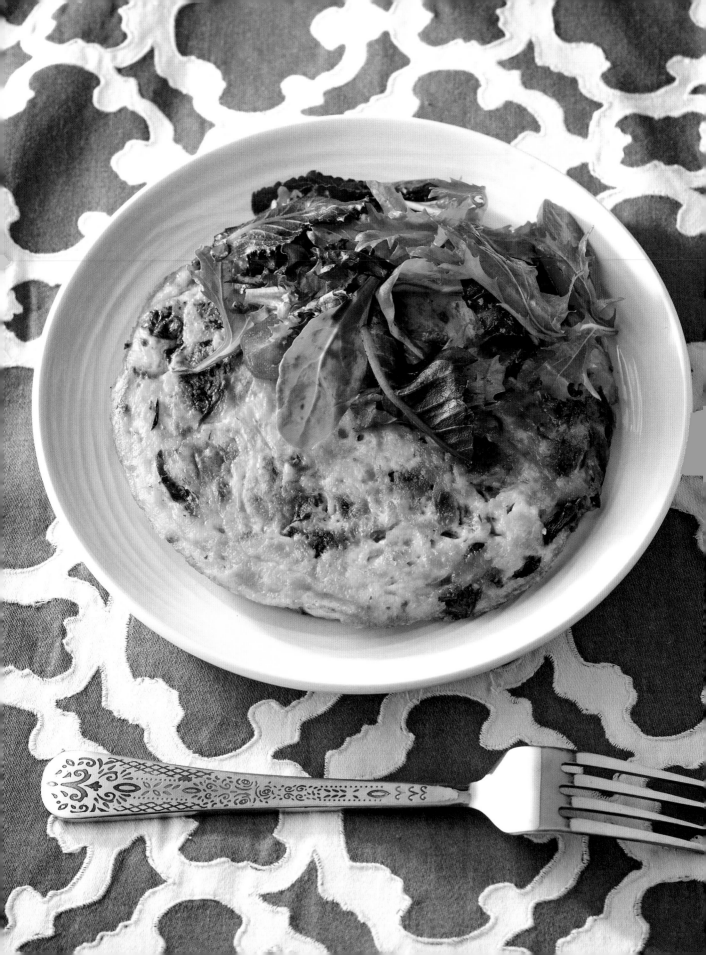

CHEESE AND LEEK FRITTATA

In my opinion, the frittata is one of the best egg dishes. Not too eggy, not at all complicated, it makes a great breakfast, lunch, or light dinner. Served with a simple salad, this dish is one of my favorite solo meals. Don't feel bound to anything but the eggs—this is a perfect meal for using up whatever is in your fridge begging for some attention (within reason, of course).

3   large eggs

2   teaspoons unsalted butter

1   teaspoon Canna-Butter (page 16)

1   small leek, cleaned well and sliced

1   cup (30 g) packed fresh spinach

¼   cup (15 g) chopped fresh Italian parsley

¼   cup (30 g) grated cheddar cheese

1. Preheat the oven to 340°F (170°C, or gas mark 3).

2. In a medium bowl, beat the eggs; set aside.

3. In a small ovenproof skillet, heat both of the butters over medium-low heat. Sauté the leek in the butter until tender, about 8 to 10 minutes. If needed to keep the pan from getting too dry, add an additional teaspoon or two of regular butter.

4. Add the spinach, parsley, and cheddar cheese to the eggs, stir to combine, and pour into the skillet. Stir a couple of times to evenly distribute the spinach and parsley before placing the pan in the oven.

5. Bake until the eggs are just set, about 15 to 20 minutes. Be careful not to overcook. Serve hot.

Yield: Serves 1

CHEF'S NOTE

When I was in cooking school, we had a day of frittata making. I had never had one before. The main lesson was: don't overcook.

CHICKEN WITH LEMON AND CAPERS

This dish can be ready in just 10 minutes. I keep chicken breasts on hand in my freezer and, when I want one for dinner, I transfer one to the fridge in the morning. By the time I'm ready for dinner, it's thawed and can be on the table in no time. I love to dip bread into this sauce. Of course I do. And I love capers, though I think they may be an acquired taste. Cannabis and capers: they're perfect together!

2   tablespoons (16 g)
    all-purpose flour

    Salt and black pepper

1   teaspoon grated lemon zest

1   boneless, skinless chicken
    breast (6 ounces, or 170 g)

2   tablespoons (28 ml) olive oil

1   teaspoon Canna-Butter
    (page 16)

    Juice of ½ of a lemon

¼   cup (60 ml) chicken broth

2   tablespoons (28 ml)
    white wine

2   teaspoons capers, drained

1   clove of garlic, minced

1. Place the flour in a plastic bag with a sprinkle of salt and black pepper and the lemon zest. Add the chicken breast to the bag and toss to coat it.

2. In a small skillet, heat the olive oil and Canna-Butter over medium-low heat. When hot, add the chicken breast and sauté for 6 to 7 minutes until cooked throughout, turning once.

3. Transfer the cooked chicken to a serving plate and cover with aluminum foil to rest while you make the sauce.

4. Add the lemon juice, chicken broth, and white wine to the skillet and simmer for 4 to 5 minutes, scraping the bottom of the pan to get all the flavorful brown bits.

5. Stir in the capers and garlic and cook for 1 minute. Remove from the heat and season with salt and black pepper to taste. Pour on top of your prepared chicken breast and enjoy!

Yield: Serves 1

CHEF'S NOTE

This dish is also great with the addition of artichoke hearts, olives, grape tomatoes, and any chopped greens you have on hand. Add these items along with the capers and garlic, if you like.

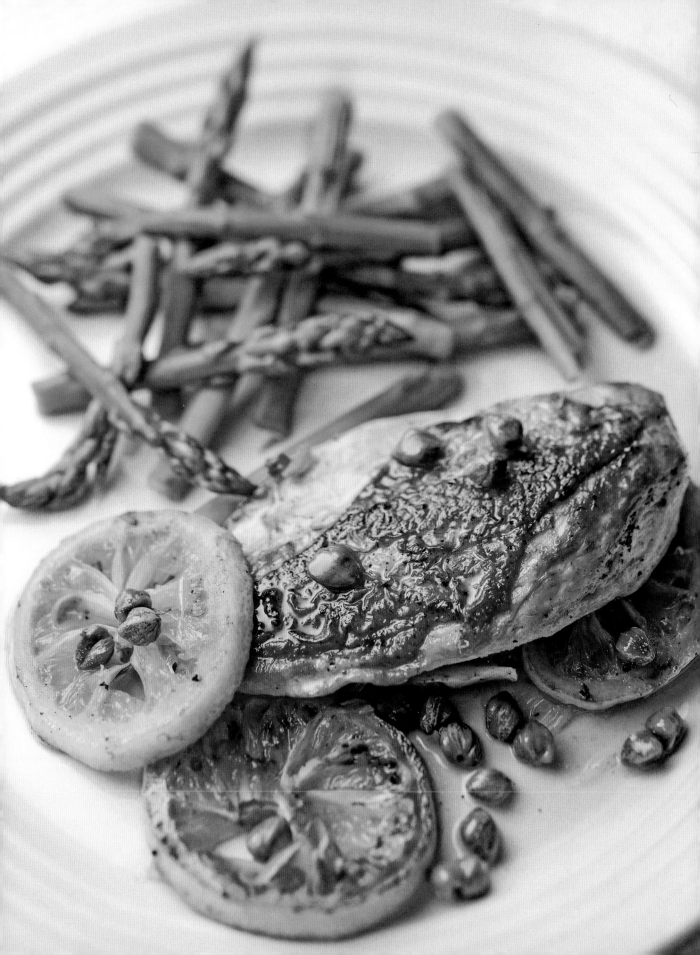

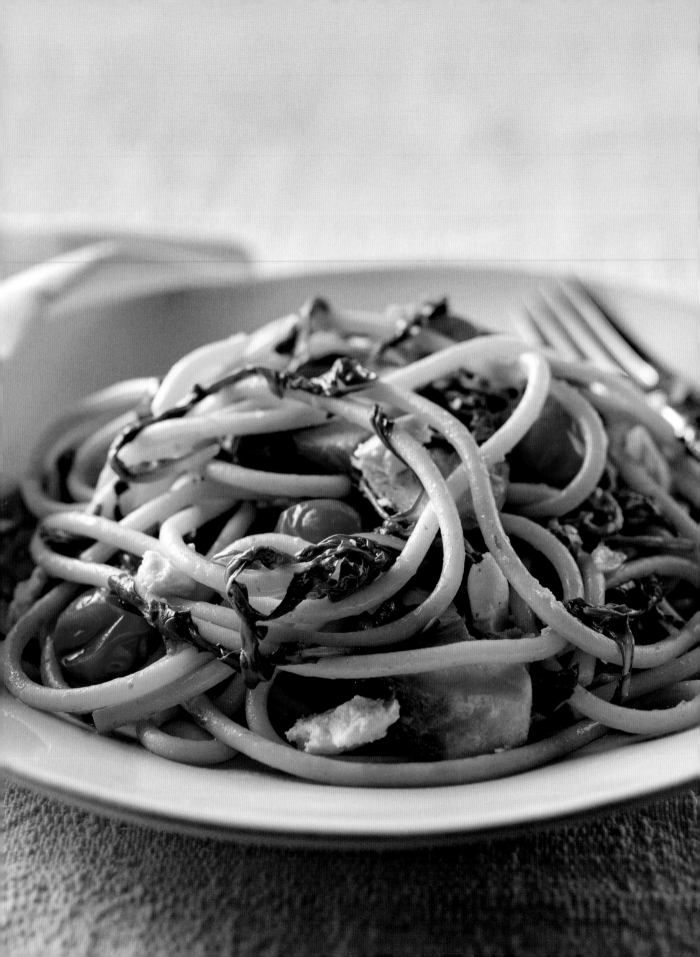

BUCATINI WITH SPINACH AND TOMATOES

Bucatini is a thick spaghetti-like pasta that is extremely satisfying. If it's not your cup of tea, feel free to use any other shape. In summertime, an angel hair pasta would be delightful. Adding cooked shrimp or chicken could also be a nice way to go.

2 tablespoons (28 ml) olive oil

1 teaspoon Canna-Oil (page 18), made with olive oil

2 cloves of garlic, sliced

4 cherry tomatoes, halved

1 cup (30 g) packed fresh spinach

   Pinch of crushed red pepper

   Salt and black pepper

3 ounces (85 g) bucatini pasta

   Grated Parmesan cheese, for garnish (optional)

1. Bring a large pot of water to a boil.

2. Meanwhile, in a medium skillet over medium-low heat, heat both of the oils. Add the garlic and cherry tomatoes and sauté for 3 to 4 minutes.

3. Add the spinach and sauté until wilted, about 3 to 4 minutes. Stir in the crushed red pepper and season with salt and black pepper to taste. Keep warm over very low heat.

4. Cook the pasta in the boiling water according to the package directions. When tender, drain and place in a bowl.

5. Add the sauce to the pasta, sprinkle with Parmesan cheese, if desired, and serve.

Yield: Serves 1

CHEF'S NOTE

Instead of sprinkling with Parmesan cheese, sauté some fresh or frozen peas along with the garlic and tomatoes and then stir in a couple of tablespoons (19 g) of goat cheese. It's an awesome flavor combination.

PARMESAN RISOTTO

The first time I had risotto was in Italy, when I was working on the cookbook of a famous chef. We traveled all over Italy, with the world's largest mortadella (an Italian sausage), and would place a plate of food in front of various beautiful locations to photograph it. It was pretty bizarre, but the food was terrific. The risotto then was as simple as this one is now. Butter and Parmesan equals Yummy.

2 teaspoons unsalted butter

1 teaspoon Canna-Butter (page 16)

1 shallot, chopped

½ cup (96 g) Arborio rice

¼ cup (60 ml) white wine

1½ cups (355 ml) chicken broth

2 tablespoons (10 g) grated Parmesan cheese, plus more for serving

Salt and coarsely ground black pepper

1. In a small saucepan over low heat, melt both of the butters. Add the shallot and cook until it softens, about 4 to 5 minutes.

2. Add the Arborio rice to the pan and stir to coat the grains for a minute or two.

3. Pour in the white wine and chicken broth and cook, stirring continuously, until the liquid is nearly absorbed, 25 to 30 minutes. Adjust the heat as needed to keep the liquid at a gentle simmer.

4. In the last few minutes of cooking, add the Parmesan cheese and stir. Season with salt and black pepper to taste. Serve with additional Parmesan cheese.

Yield: Serves 1

CHEF'S NOTE

If you like a creamier risotto, add another ¼ cup (60 ml) of chicken broth or water. If you want to add some visual and flavor interest to the dish, add some cooked and chopped bacon or pancetta and some chopped sun-dried tomatoes to the risotto when you stir in the Parmesan cheese.

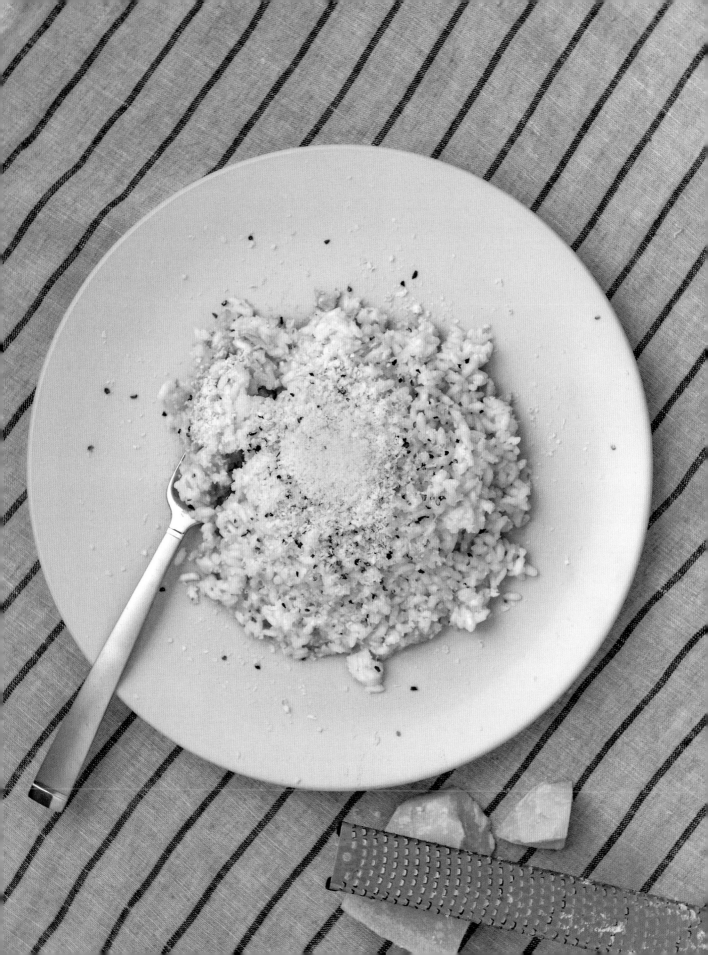

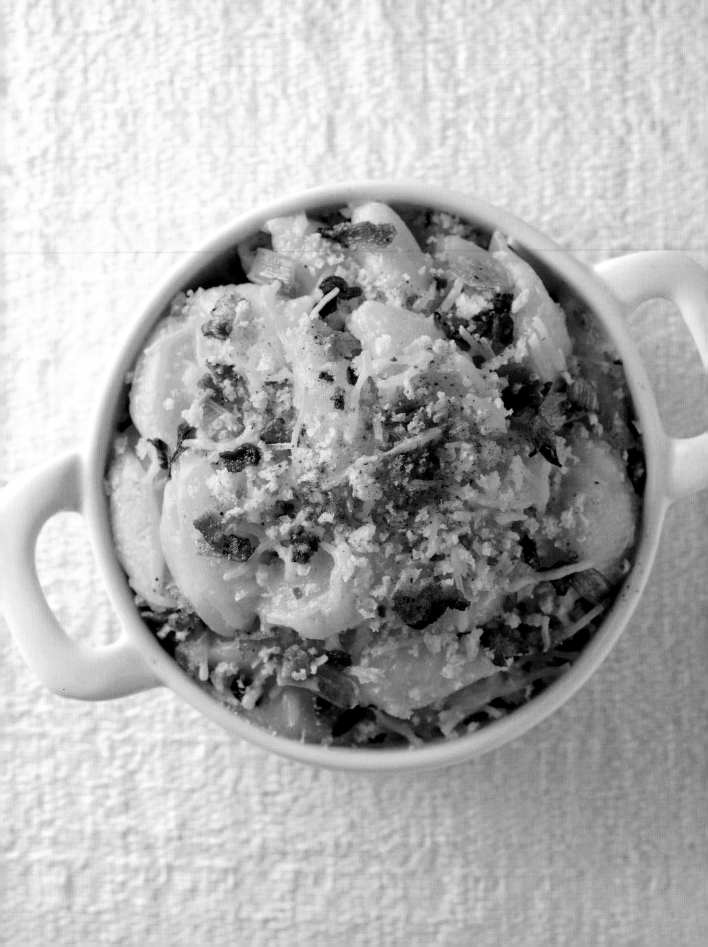

BACON MAC AND CHEESE

There's no reason that mac and cheese has to be a dish for a big crowd—it's perfect for just one person. When you're home alone and a craving for the ultimate comfort food hits, this recipe will make you one serving of cheesy bliss.

2 teaspoons unsalted butter, plus 1 tablespoon (14 g), melted

1 teaspoon Canna-Butter (page 16)

1 tablespoon (8 g) all-purpose flour

¼ teaspoon salt

Pinch of black pepper

½ cup (120 ml) milk (whole or 2%)

½ cup (58 g) shredded cheddar cheese

½ teaspoon dry mustard

½ teaspoon Worcestershire sauce

2 strips of bacon, cooked, drained, and chopped

2 scallions, chopped

¼ cup (23 g) small pasta, cooked and drained

2 tablespoons (8 g) panko bread crumbs

Paprika, for garnish

1. Preheat the oven to 340°F (170°C, or gas mark 3). Spray an 8-ounce (235 ml) baking dish with a light coating of cooking spray. Set aside.

2. In a medium nonstick skillet, heat the 2 teaspoons butter and the Canna-Butter over medium-low heat. Stir to combine. Add the flour, salt, and black pepper, whisking to incorporate. Continue to whisk until the flour begins to turn a light golden color, about 3 to 4 minutes. Gradually add the milk, whisking continuously. While stirring, cook for 6 to 7 minutes until the sauce begins to thicken. Remove from the heat.

3. Stir in the cheddar cheese, dry mustard, Worcestershire sauce, bacon, scallions, and cooked pasta and place in the prepared baking dish.

4. In a small bowl, combine the panko bread crumbs with the melted butter and sprinkle on top of the macaroni mixture.

5. Dust with paprika. Bake until golden brown and bubbling, about 12 to 15 minutes. Serve hot.

Yield: Serves 1

CHICKEN MILANESE WITH FRESH SALSA

The crunch of the cutlet with this topping is pretty memorable. If you don't feel like doing a lot of chopping, you can top the chicken with a simple salad of your favorite greens, lightly dressed. I am kind of ashamed to say I am not much of a salad person, but this dish is pretty dreamy. This recipe also works well with a pounded pork cutlet.

½ of a Roma tomato, chopped

¼ of a yellow bell pepper, chopped

1 radish, chopped

2 tablespoons (12 g) thinly sliced scallion

2 tablespoons (8 g) chopped fresh Italian parsley

2 tablespoons chopped avocado, tossed with the juice of ½ of a lemon

2 tablespoons (28 ml) olive oil

1 teaspoon Canna-Oil (page 18), made with olive oil

Juice of ½ of a lemon

Salt and black pepper

1 large egg, lightly beaten

½ cup (30 g) panko bread crumbs

¼ cup (25 g) grated Parmesan cheese

2 tablespoons (28 ml) canola oil

1 boneless, skinless chicken breast, pounded thin

1. In a small bowl, combine the tomato, bell pepper, radish, scallion, 1 tablespoon (4 g) of the parsley, and the avocado.

2. Add both of the oils and the lemon juice and season with salt and black pepper to taste. Toss well and chill until ready to serve.

3. Place the beaten egg in a shallow bowl. On a plate, combine the panko bread crumbs, Parmesan cheese, and remaining 1 tablespoon (4 g) parsley.

4. In a medium skillet, heat the canola oil.

5. Dip the chicken breast into the egg, followed by the bread crumb mixture, and then carefully place it in the hot skillet.

6. Cook the chicken breast in the oil until cooked throughout and the crust is crisp, about 4 minutes per side.

7. Transfer to a plate and top with the salsa. Serve immediately.

Yield: Serves 1

CHEF'S NOTE In this dish, you want the contrast of the hot chicken and the cool vegetable topping. So be sure to make and chill the salsa before you cook the chicken. You can even make it the night before, but just add the avocado as close to dinner as possible so that it doesn't turn brown.

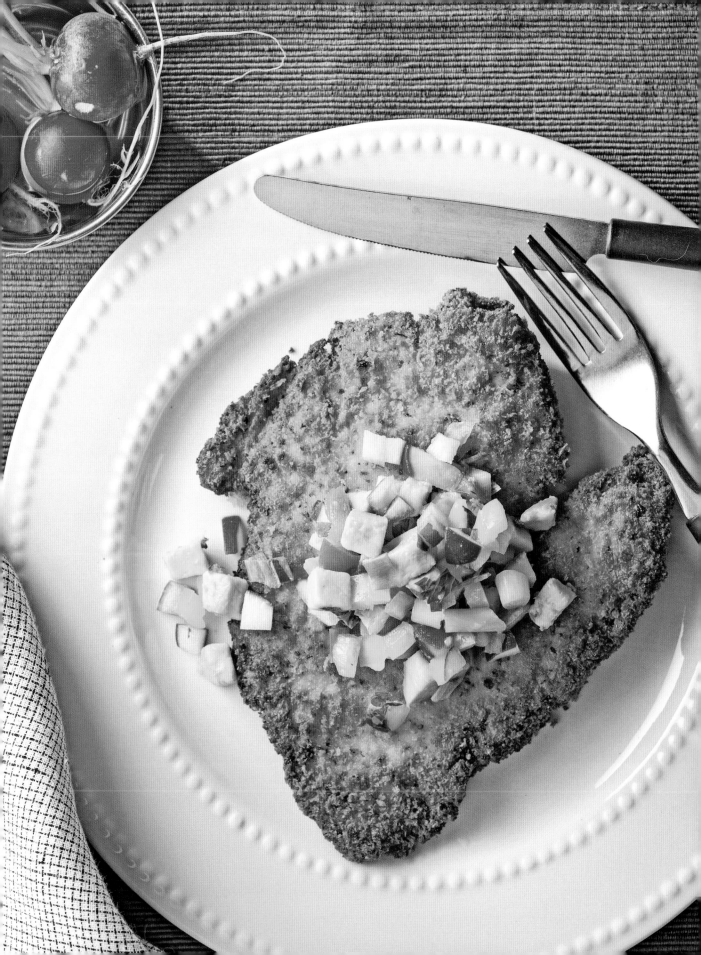

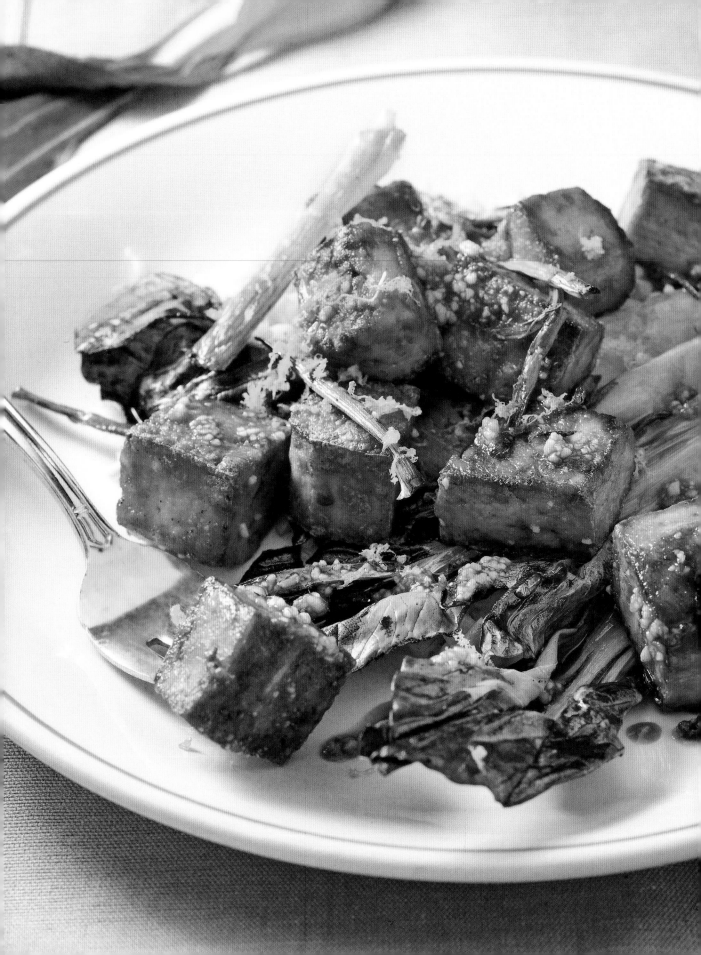

SEARED AND BAKED SESAME TOFU WITH PEANUT SAUCE

Tofu is kind of a blank slate. It has almost no flavor by itself, but it beautifully absorbs whatever flavors you have in mind for it. I like to let it marinate for about 30 minutes before cooking. The searing does wonders for the texture, which in my opinion is pretty abysmal without any help.

½ of a 14-ounce block (390 g) extra-firm tofu, cubed

2 tablespoons (28 ml) soy sauce

1 tablespoon (15 ml) rice vinegar

1 tablespoon (15 ml) toasted sesame oil

1 teaspoon grated fresh ginger

1 teaspoon honey

1 head of bok choy

1 teaspoon canola oil

2 tablespoons (32 g) peanut butter

1 teaspoon Canna-Oil (page 18), made with canola oil

½ teaspoon soy sauce

1 scallion, chopped

Zest of ½ of an orange

1. Preheat the oven to 400°F (200°C, or gas mark 6).

2. In a medium bowl, combine the tofu with the soy sauce, rice vinegar, sesame oil, ginger, and honey. Allow to marinate for 30 minutes.

3. Toss the bok choy with the canola oil. Place the tofu and the bok choy on a rimmed baking sheet. Roast, turning the tofu a couple of times, for 25 to 30 minutes, until golden brown and slightly crispy.

4. In a small bowl, combine the peanut butter, Canna-Oil, and soy sauce. Toss with the tofu and sprinkle with the chopped scallion and orange zest. Serve hot.

Yield: Serves 1

CHEF'S NOTE If you are using tofu that is not extra-firm, you may want to press the moisture out before cooking. Place on a clean kitchen towel and weigh down with a pan for 10 to 15 minutes to press out the excess moisture.

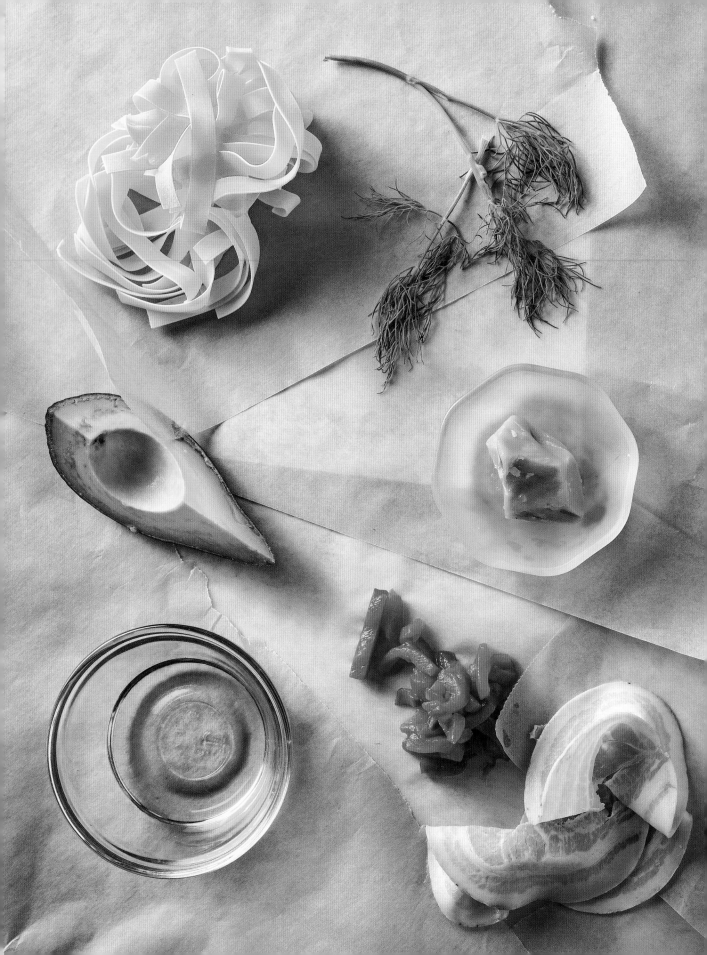

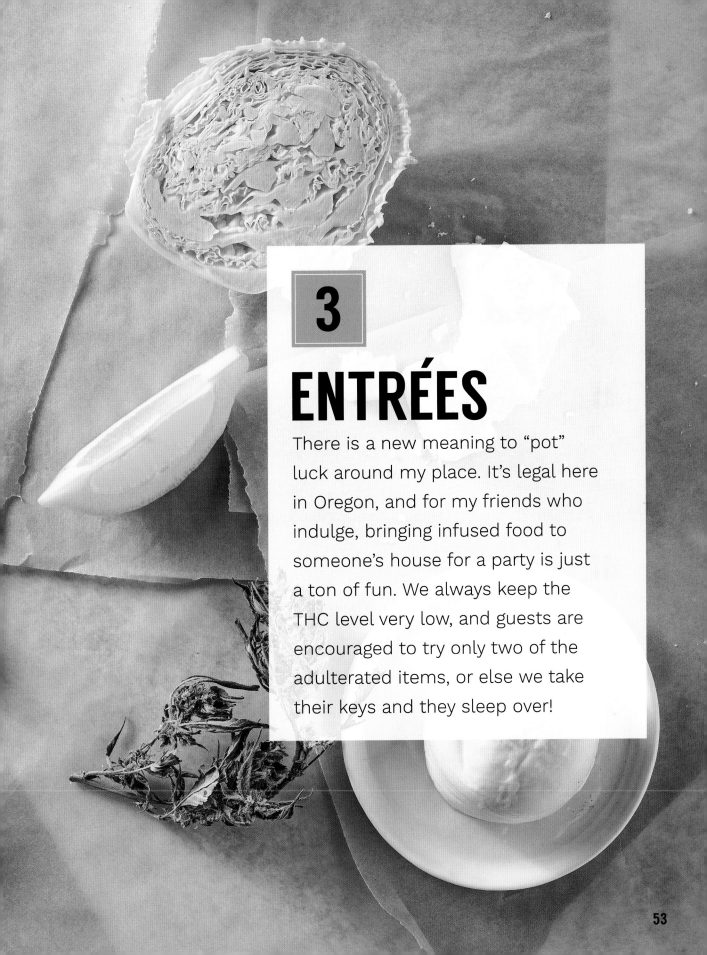

3

ENTRÉES

There is a new meaning to "pot" luck around my place. It's legal here in Oregon, and for my friends who indulge, bringing infused food to someone's house for a party is just a ton of fun. We always keep the THC level very low, and guests are encouraged to try only two of the adulterated items, or else we take their keys and they sleep over!

MEATBALLS IN MARINARA

I love a good meatball. Cocktail, Swedish, turkey, pork . . . a well-made meatball always hits the spot. I like to sauté the onion and garlic in the Canna-Oil before mixing them with the other ingredients. These meatballs are very flavorful, and I think they might even taste better the day after they're made. And they freeze well, too. Serve over cooked ziti.

MEATBALLS

2 tablespoons (28 ml) Canna-Oil (page 18), made with olive oil

1 large onion, finely chopped

2 cloves of garlic, minced

1 pound (455 g) ground beef

½ pound (225 g) ground pork

2 large eggs

1 cup (100 g) grated Parmesan cheese, plus more for garnish

1 cup (115 g) bread crumbs

¼ cup (15 g) chopped fresh Italian parsley

½ cup (120 ml) milk

Salt and black pepper

MARINARA SAUCE

3 tablespoons (45 ml) olive oil

1 large yellow onion, diced

3 cloves of garlic, minced

3 tablespoons (48 g) tomato paste

3 cans (28 ounces, or 785 g) plum tomatoes

1 cup (235 ml) water

1 tablespoon (15 ml) balsamic vinegar

Salt and black pepper

1. <u>To make the meatballs:</u> In a large sauté pan, heat the Canna-Oil over low heat. Sauté the onion and garlic until translucent, about 5 to 7 minutes.

2. Combine the onion-garlic mixture with the rest of the meatball ingredients in a large bowl, being sure to distribute the ingredients evenly throughout the mixture. Place in the refrigerator while you prepare the sauce.

3. <u>To make the marinara sauce:</u> Heat the olive oil in a large saucepan over low heat. Sauté the onion and garlic until translucent, about 5 to 7 minutes. Add the tomato paste and sauté for 2 to 3 minutes.

4. Add the cans of tomatoes and the water, stir, cover, and cook for 2 to 3 hours, stirring occasionally. The sauce will get thicker and richer the longer it cooks.

5. Add the balsamic vinegar and season with salt and black pepper to taste.

6. Remove the meatball mixture from the refrigerator and form into eighteen 2-inch (5 cm) balls. Drop the balls into the sauce and cook for 2 to 3 hours until the meatballs are fully cooked. Store leftovers in an airtight container in the refrigerator for up to 5 days or the freezer for up to 3 months.

Yield: Serves 6 (3 meatballs per serving)

CHEF'S NOTE Making a meatball sub with mozzarella cheese could be the tastiest way to handle leftovers.

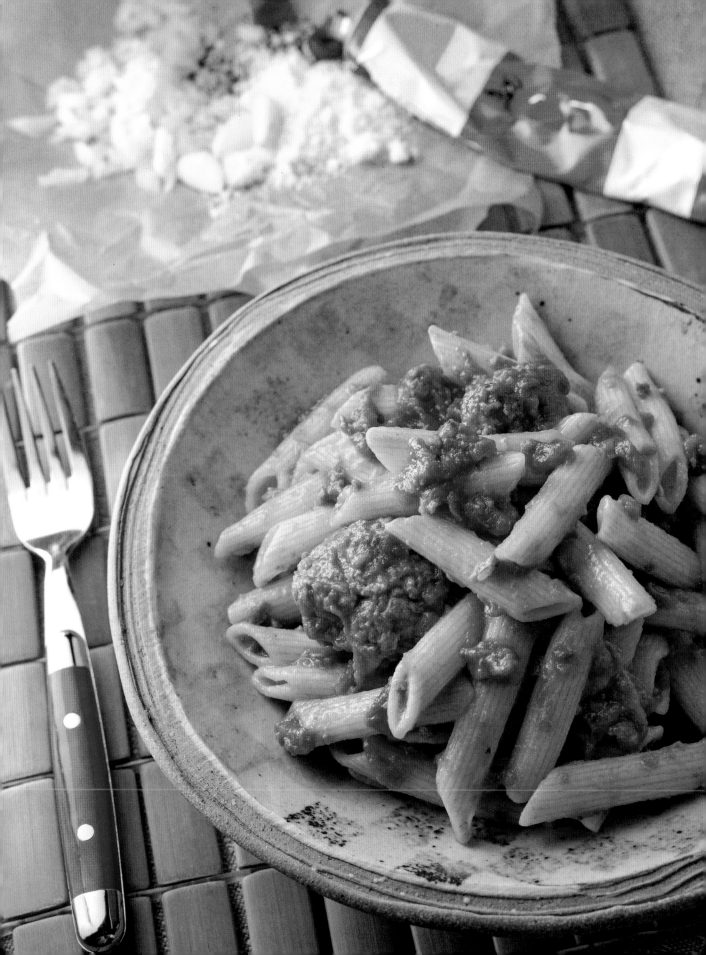

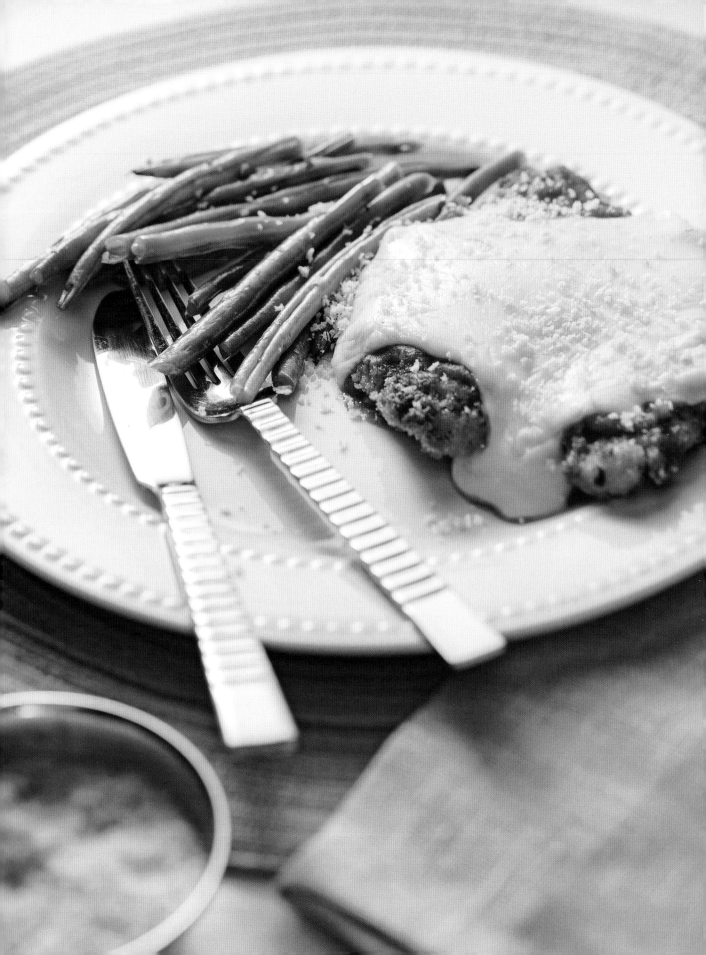

CHICKEN PARMESAN

When I was growing up in the Bronx, we made a weekly pilgrimage to a restaurant that had amazing chicken Parmesan, which would arrive at the table bubbling in a metal dish. It was perfect. This recipe is pretty close, no metal dish required. Any leftover sauce will freeze beautifully.

MARINARA SAUCE

- 3 tablespoons (45 ml) olive oil
- 1 large yellow onion, diced
- 3 cloves of garlic, minced
- 3 tablespoons (48 g) tomato paste
- 3 cans (28 ounces, or 785 g, each) plum tomatoes
- 1 cup (235 ml) water
- Balsamic vinegar
- Salt and black pepper

CHICKEN

- 1 large egg, lightly beaten
- ½ cup (60 g) bread crumbs
- ¼ cup (25 g) grated Parmesan cheese, plus more for garnish
- Salt and black pepper
- 2 boneless, skinless chicken breasts
- 2 tablespoons (28 g) canola oil
- 2 teaspoons Canna-Oil (page 18)
- 2 cloves of garlic, minced
- 4 to 6 slices of good-quality mozzarella cheese

1. Preheat the oven to 340°F (170°C, or gas mark 3).

2. To make the marinara sauce: Heat the olive oil in a large saucepan over low heat. Sauté the onion and garlic until translucent, about 5 to 7 minutes. Add the tomato paste and sauté for 2 to 3 minutes.

3. Add the cans of tomatoes and the water, stir, cover, and cook for 2 to 3 hours, stirring occasionally.

4. Remove from the heat, add the balsamic vinegar, and season with salt and black pepper to taste.

5. To make the chicken: In a medium bowl, beat the egg. Mix the bread crumbs, Parmesan cheese, and salt and black pepper to taste on a plate. Dip the chicken first in the egg and then in the bread crumbs.

6. Heat both of the oils in a large skillet over medium heat. Add the garlic and sauté for 1 minute. Place the chicken breasts in the pan and cook on one side till golden brown, about 4 to 5 minutes, and then turn and cook on the other side for another 4 to 5 minutes. Drain on paper towels.

7. Place the chicken breasts in a 9-inch (23 cm) square baking dish. Pour the sauce over the chicken and top with the slices of mozzarella cheese.

8. Bake until the cheese is melted and the sauce is bubbling, about 25 to 30 minutes. Serve hot.

Yield: Serves 2

 CHEF'S NOTE With chicken Parmesan, you can use either a regular chicken breast or one that has been pounded thin. You can usually ask the butcher, even in a supermarket, to do the pounding for you.

SPAGHETTI CARBONARA

Everyone should know how to make pasta carbonara. It's easy and takes just a few minutes to create a wonderful dish!

2   tablespoons (28 ml) olive oil

4   teaspoons (20 ml) Canna-Oil (page 18), made with olive oil

2   ounces (55 g) pancetta or lardons of bacon, cut into small pieces

2   cloves of garlic, finely chopped

3   large eggs

½   cup (50 g) grated Parmesan cheese, plus more for garnish

1   pound (455 g) spaghetti

Salt and black pepper

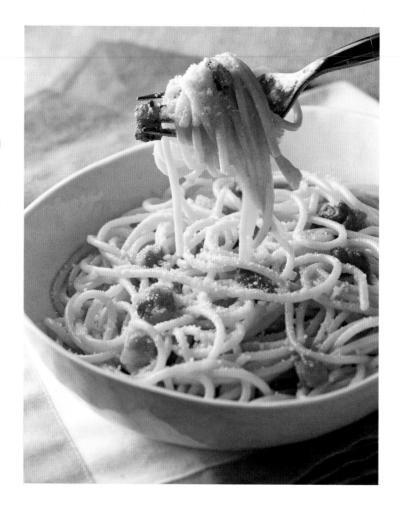

1. In a large sauté pan, heat both of the oils over medium-low heat. Add the pancetta and cook for 2 to 3 minutes until it is starting to get crispy around the edges. Add the garlic and sauté for 1 minute. Keep warm over low heat.

2. In a medium bowl, whisk the eggs with the Parmesan cheese, stirring well to remove any lumps.

3. Bring a large pot of water to a boil and cook the pasta according to the package directions. The pasta needs to be hot for this dish to be successful. Drain the pasta and add to the pan with the pancetta and oil.

4. Remove the pan from the heat and add the egg mixture to the pasta. Whisk quickly to combine, as you do not want the eggs to scramble, but rather just coat the strands of spaghetti in a silky sauce.

5. Season with salt and black pepper to taste, sprinkle with Parmesan cheese, and serve immediately.

Yield: Serves 4

PORK WITH CABBAGE AND APPLES

If you're careful not to overcook the pork cutlet here, you'll be rewarded with a very tasty dish. The apples and cabbage add crunch and sweetness, making the dish both satisfying and light.

2   **boneless pork cutlets (10 ounces, or 280 g)**

½   **teaspoon salt**

½   **teaspoon black pepper**

2   **tablespoons (28 ml) olive oil**

1   **apple, cored and sliced into wedges**

¼   **of a head of savoy cabbage, shredded**

3   **scallions, cut into pieces**

2   **tablespoons (28 ml) maple syrup**

2   **teaspoons Canna-Butter (page 16)**

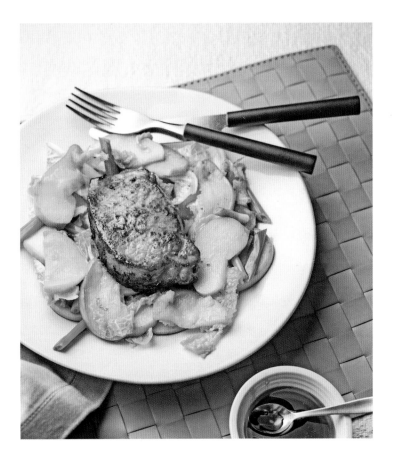

1. Place the pork cutlets on your work surface. Season with the salt and black pepper.

2. In a large skillet over medium heat, heat the olive oil and sauté the apple and cabbage until tender, about 5 to 7 minutes. Transfer to a plate.

3. Return the pan to the heat and sauté the pork cutlets for 4 minutes on each side until golden brown.

4. Return the vegetables to the skillet and add the scallions. Cook for 2 to 3 minutes. Add the maple syrup and Canna-Butter and stir to mix well. Taste and season with salt and black pepper as desired and serve.

Yield: Serves 2

CHEF'S NOTE The recommended cooking temperature for these chops is 145°F (63°C). Pork can be pink in the center and still safe to eat. And it's delicious.

BACON-TOPPED MEATLOAF

Perhaps one of the best comfort foods, meatloaf gets a bad rap. My father would only eat meatloaf if it had bacon on it. I will only eat it if it has cannabis in it! That's not true, actually: I love my meatloaf too much to turn away the cannabis-free variety. But with a bacon topping and cannabis, this may just be the greatest meatloaf ever.

3 tablespoons (45 ml) Canna-Oil (page 18), made with olive oil

1 large yellow onion, chopped

2 cloves of garlic, minced

1½ pounds (680 g) ground beef

½ pound (225 g) ground pork

1 cup (50 g) fresh bread crumbs

½ cup (120 ml) milk

⅔ cup (160 g) ketchup

2 teaspoons Worcestershire sauce

1 teaspoon salt

Freshly ground black pepper

6 strips of bacon, cut in half crosswise

1. Preheat the oven to 340°F (170°C, or gas mark 3).

2. In a large sauté pan over medium heat, heat the Canna-Oil. Sauté the onion and garlic for 4 to 5 minutes until translucent.

3. In a large bowl, combine the beef, pork, bread crumbs, milk, ketchup, Worcestershire sauce, salt, and black pepper. Add the onion and garlic mixture and mix to combine thoroughly.

4. Transfer the mixture to a 9-inch (23 cm) loaf pan. Top with the bacon slices.

5. Bake the meatloaf for about 60 minutes. The bacon will be crispy on top, the meat will be browned, and the interior temperature of the meatloaf should be 155°F (68°C). Store leftovers in an airtight container in the refrigerator for up to 5 days.

Yield: Serves 9

CHEF'S NOTE Make your leftover meatloaf into meatloaf sandwiches. Spread some mayo (regular or Canna-Mayonnaise, page 20), Dijon mustard, and maybe ketchup on two slices of bread and top with your sliced meatloaf, lettuce, and onion. Pickle slices add a great crunchy tang.

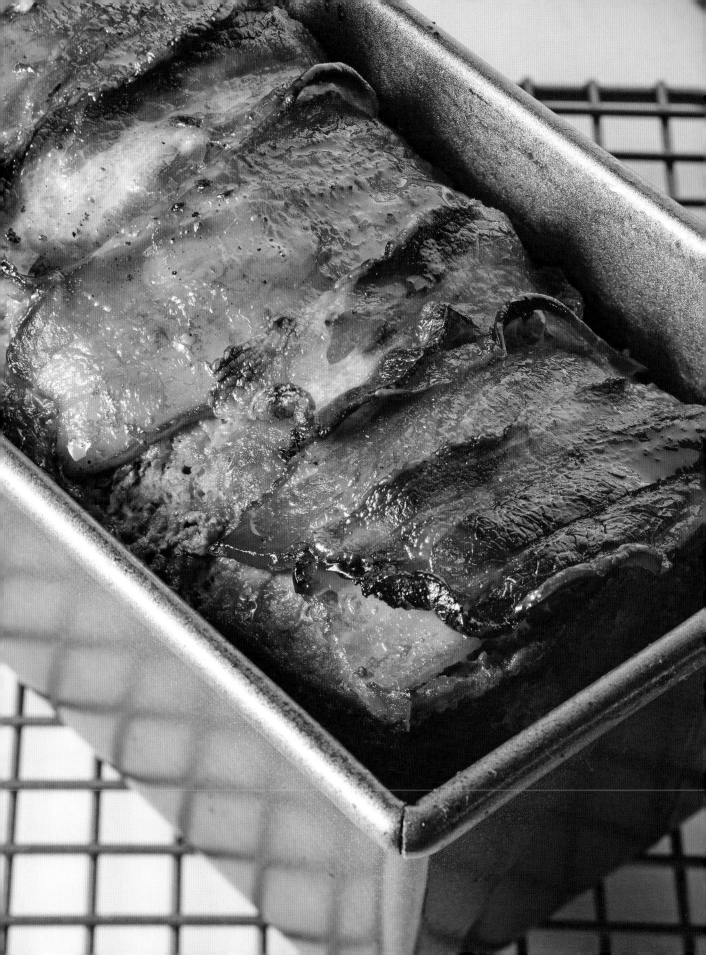

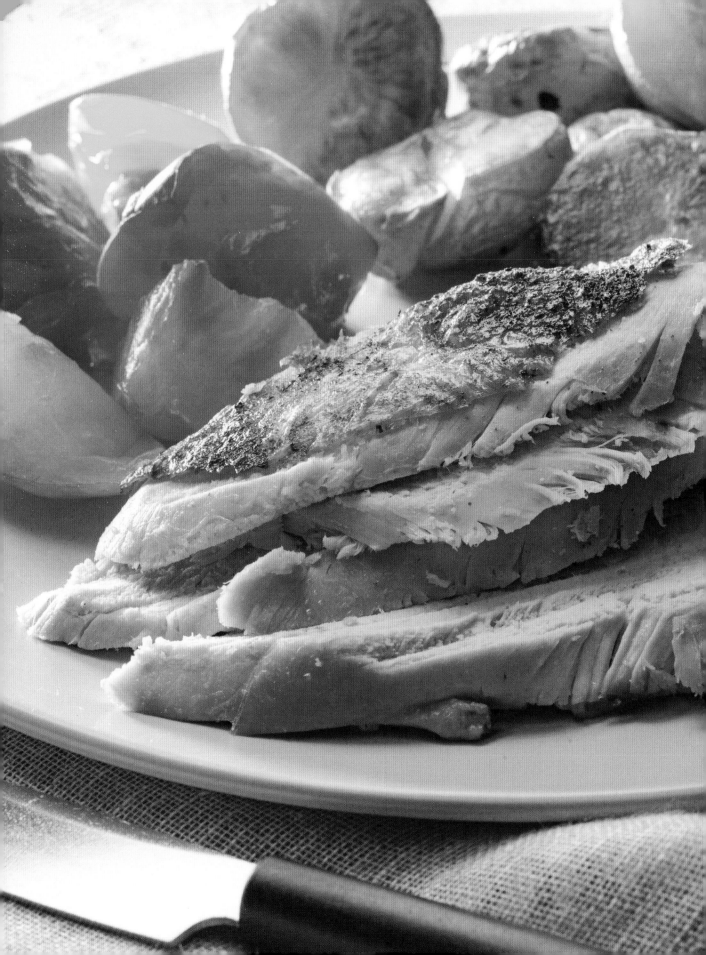

ROAST CHICKEN

Once I tasted the combination of chicken and smoked paprika, I was hooked. The earthy notes from the cannabis and smoked paprika are also great together. So this chicken with paprika and cannabis proves to be a fantastic combination. I like the cannabis to peek through in this dish, becoming its own flavorful herb.

1   **roasting chicken (5 to 6 pounds, or 2.3 to 2.7 kg)**

2   **tablespoons (28 ml) olive oil**

    Salt and black pepper

1   **large carrot, peeled and cut into large pieces**

1   **medium yellow onion, peeled and cut into chunks**

1   **orange, cut into wedges**

1   **head of garlic, top cut off**

2   **tablespoons (28 g) Canna-Butter (page 16)**

2   **tablespoons (16 g) all-purpose flour**

2   **cups (475 ml) chicken broth**

1   **teaspoon smoked paprika**

1. Preheat over to 340°F (170°C, or gas mark 3).

2. Place the chicken on your work surface. Rub with the olive oil and season with salt and black pepper all over. Place in a roasting pan.

3. Place half of the carrot, onion, and orange pieces inside of the chicken cavity and place the rest of the pieces in the pan, along with the head of garlic.

4. Roast the chicken for 90 minutes or until the juices from the thigh area run clear and an instant-read thermometer inserted into the thigh without touching bone reads 165°F (74°C). Transfer the chicken to a plate and discard the vegetables from the pan.

5. Heat the Canna-Butter in the roasting pan on the stove over medium heat. When hot, add the flour, stirring constantly. Cook for 2 minutes and then add the chicken broth and smoked paprika and cook for 4 to 5 minutes until the sauce thickens.

6. Taste and adjust the seasoning with salt and black pepper. Pour the sauce into a gravy boat or serving vessel of choice. Carve the chicken into serving pieces and place on a platter. Store leftovers in an airtight container in the refrigerator for up to 5 days.

Yield: Serves 6

CHEF'S NOTE Roast chicken is one of those elemental foods that you really need to know how to cook. It's versatile, has great leftover options, and offers such great flavor. And when the meat is all gone, let there be soup. Save the bones to make a wonderful homemade stock.

CHICKEN POT PIES

If you use store-bought piecrust or puff pastry, this is an easy way to enjoy an infused comfort food classic. Just the thought of breaking through the top crust is enough to give me goose bumps. If you have only ever had a frozen version of this chicken pot pie, you are in for a treat.

3   **tablespoons (42 g) unsalted butter**

4   **teaspoons (19 g) Canna-Butter (page 16)**

1   **stalk of celery, sliced**

1   **carrot, peeled and sliced**

1   **teaspoon fresh thyme leaves**

⅓   **cup (42 g) all-purpose flour**

2   **cups (475 ml) chicken broth**

⅓   **cup (80 ml) half-and-half or Canna-Cream (page 24)**

1   **cup (150 g) fresh or (130 g) frozen green peas**

3   **cups (420 g) cooked and chopped chicken**

    Salt and black pepper

1   **box puff pastry (1 pound, or 455 g) or double-crust piecrust, thawed if necessary**

1   **large egg, beaten (optional)**

1. In a large sauté pan over low heat, melt both of the butters. Sauté the celery, carrot, and thyme for 10 minutes or until the vegetables are softened.

2. Add the flour to the mixture and cook for 2 minutes, stirring occasionally. Add the chicken broth, half-and-half, and peas and mix well until the vegetables are coated and the mixture starts to thicken. Stir in the chicken. Season with salt and black pepper to taste.

3. Preheat the oven to 340°F (170°C, or gas mark 3).

4. Roll out the pastry dough and then cut the pastry to fit the tops of four 8-ounce (235 ml) ramekins.

5. Divide the chicken mixture among the ramekins and top with the pastry. If desired, brush the pastry with the beaten egg for a shiny, crisp crust. Make slits in the pastry with a sharp knife to let the steam escape.

6. Bake for 25 to 30 minutes until the crust is golden brown and the filling mixture is bubbling.

Yield: Serves 4

CHEF'S NOTE

There are many versions of savory pot pie. Once for a New Year's Eve dinner, I made a lobster pot pie, which was extraordinary—and extraordinarily expensive. Chicken is the classic for a reason, and it is the way forward toward experimentation.

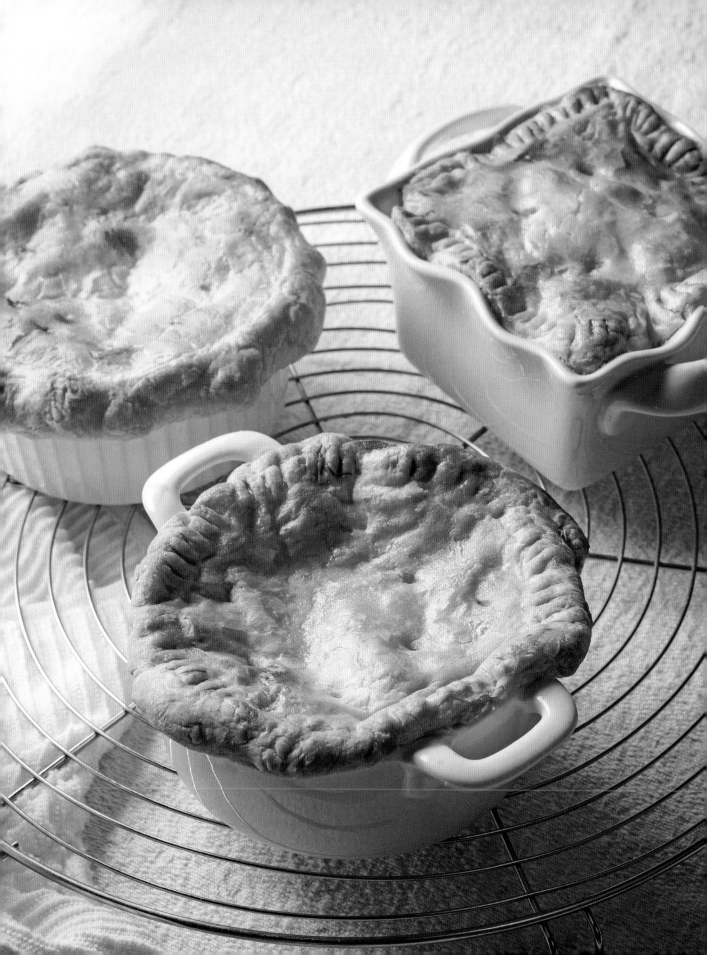

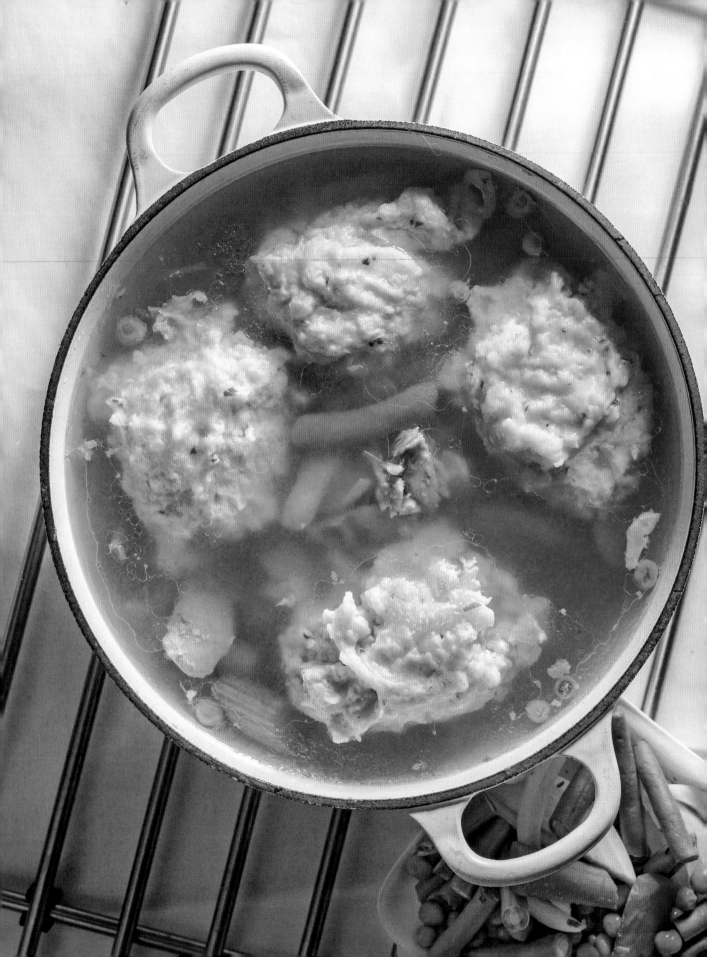

CHICKEN STEW WITH DUMPLINGS

At my good friend Lisa Schroeder's restaurant in Portland, Mother's Bistro, she serves an amazing chicken with dumplings. Her dish inspired me to create this infused recipe. The dumplings in this dish have a lot of flavor, with just a hint of cannabis, and are fluffy perfection.

STEW

6   chicken thighs (1 pound, or 455 g), skin removed

6   cups (1.4 L) chicken broth

1   stalk of celery, sliced

1   large carrot, peeled and cut into pieces

      Salt and ground black pepper

¼   pound (115 g) green beans, trimmed and cut into pieces

⅔   cup (100 g) fresh or (87 g) frozen green peas

DUMPLINGS

1½   cups (188 g) all-purpose flour

2   teaspoons baking powder

½   teaspoon salt

¼   teaspoon black pepper

1   large egg

⅔   cup (160 ml) milk

4   teaspoons (19 g) Canna-Butter (page 16)

1   tablespoon (4 g) finely chopped fresh dill

1   tablespoon (4 g) finely chopped fresh Italian parsley

1. To make the stew: In a large soup pot, combine the chicken thighs, chicken broth, celery, and carrot, and salt and black pepper, and cook over medium heat until the chicken is done, about 1 hour. The juices should run clear when the skin is pierced with a knife. Occasionally skim the foam from the top of the soup.

2. Remove the chicken from the pot and, when cool enough to handle, take the meat off the bones. Return the meat to the pot. Add the green beans and peas to the pot and simmer for 10 minutes.

3. To make the dumplings: In a large bowl, combine the flour, baking powder, salt, and black pepper. Stir in the egg, milk, Canna-Butter, dill, and parsley. Form into 8 balls.

4. Place the dumplings on the top of the soup and cover. Cook for 12 minutes and then uncover and cook for an additional 10 minutes. Taste and adjust the seasoning with salt and black pepper. Store leftovers in an airtight container in the refrigerator for up to 4 days.

Yield: Serves 4

CHEF'S NOTE Mix the dumpling dough until just combined. Don't overwork the dough or the dumplings will become tough.

SALMON WITH ROASTED RED PEPPER PUREE

Salmon and basil are a great flavor combination. When making the red pepper sauce for this dish, I always try to roast my bell peppers from scratch, but using jarred roasted red peppers will also work well. Just sauté them for a minute or two before pureeing. This dish has such a pretty color palette and such great taste.

4   salmon fillets (6 ounces, or 170 g, each)

1   tablespoon (15 ml) olive oil
     Salt and black pepper

4   teaspoons (20 ml) Canna-Oil (page 18), made with olive oil

3   roasted red bell peppers, cut into strips

¼   cup (40 g) chopped yellow onion

2   cloves of garlic, minced

1   cup (235 ml) chicken broth

¼   cup (60 ml) Canna-Cream (page 24) or heavy cream (optional)

12   small bell peppers (any color), cut in half and seeded

⅓   cup (87 g) prepared pesto
     Chopped fresh basil or Italian parsley, for garnish

1. Preheat the oven to 425°F (220°C, or gas mark 7).

2. Place the salmon on a rimmed baking sheet. Brush with the olive oil and sprinkle with salt and black pepper.

3. In a medium sauté pan over medium heat, heat the Canna-Oil. Sauté the red bell pepper strips, onion, and garlic until the onion is soft, about 4 to 5 minutes.

4. In a blender or food processor, combine the red bell pepper mixture with the chicken broth and the Canna-Cream, if using. Taste and adjust the seasoning with salt and black pepper. Return the red bell pepper mixture to the sauté pan over low heat to keep warm.

5. Place the small bell peppers on your work surface. Spoon a teaspoon of pesto into the halved peppers. Arrange on the baking sheet around the salmon. Roast the salmon and stuffed peppers in the oven and until just cooked through, about 12 to 15 minutes.

6. Transfer the salmon to plates. Add 3 stuffed pepper halves and spoon the red bell pepper sauce over the salmon. Garnish with the fresh herbs and serve.

Yield: Serves 4

CHEF'S NOTE

When roasting the salmon, please don't overcook it. A little underdone in the center is the way to go.

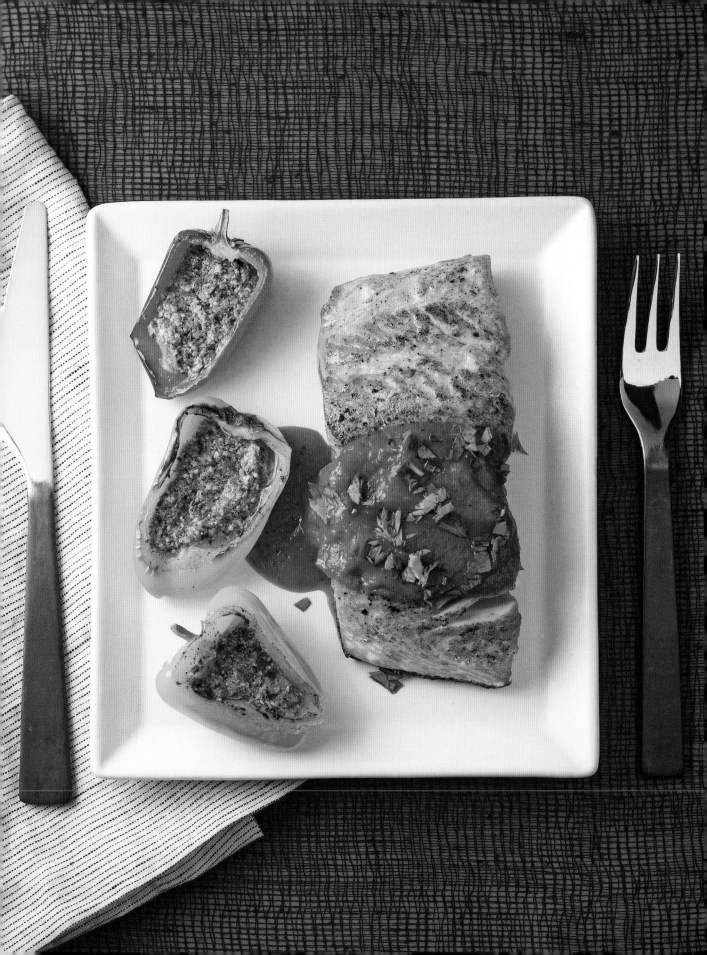

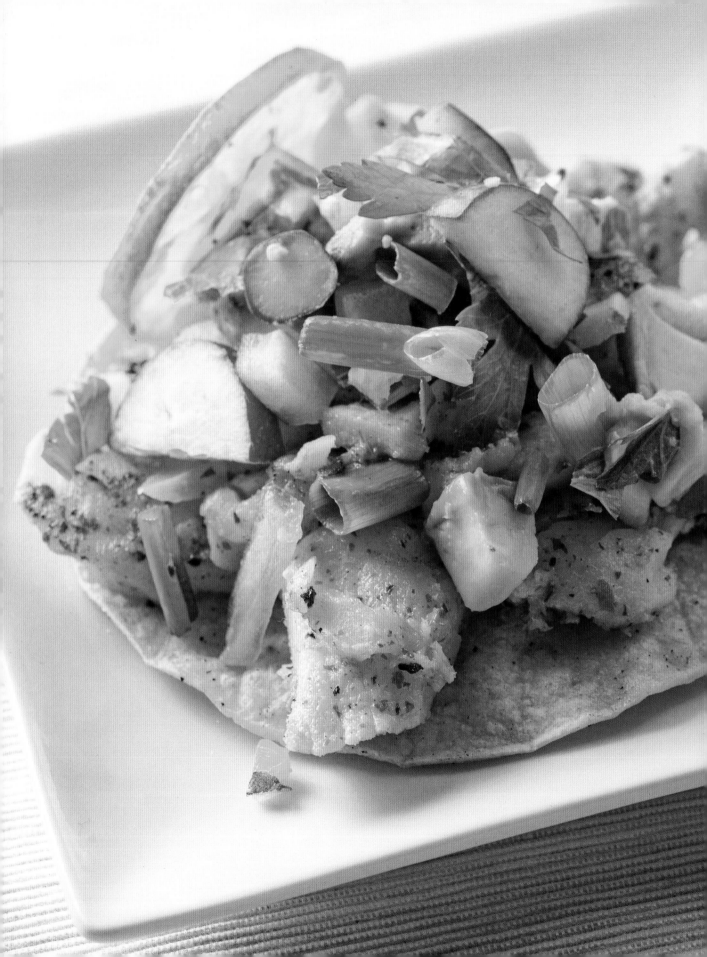

FISH TACOS

I can't resist giving the tortillas a quick fry since it makes them so delightfully crunchy. I use Pacific cod in these tacos, which is softer and flakier (and more sustainable) than Atlantic cod, and the flavor holds up well to the herbs and spices. But you can use any flaky white fish.

¼   **cup (60 ml) canola oil**

8   **small flour tortillas**

4   **radishes, thinly sliced**

3   **scallions, sliced**

½   **of a yellow bell pepper, cut into chunks**

½   **of an avocado, peeled, cubed, and tossed with lemon juice**

2   **tablespoons (20 g) chopped red onion**

2   **cloves of garlic, minced**

½   **pound (225 g) cod**

     Salt and black pepper

4   **teaspoons (20 ml) Canna-Oil (page 18), made with olive oil**

1   **tablespoon (15 ml) olive oil**

     Fresh cilantro or Italian parsley leaves, for garnish

     Lemon slices, for garnish

1. In a medium saucepan over medium heat, heat the canola oil. Quickly sauté the tortillas for a minute or two per side. Drain on paper towels.

2. In a medium bowl, combine the radishes, scallions, yellow bell pepper, avocado, red onion, and garlic. Set aside.

3. Place the fish on your work surface. Sprinkle with salt and black pepper. In a medium saucepan over medium-high heat, heat the Canna-Oil and olive oil. Break the fish into pieces and sauté quickly, about 3 to 4 minutes.

4. Add the fish to the vegetable mixture in the bowl, tossing gently to combine.

5. Place 2 tortillas on each plate. Top each tortilla with some of the fish mixture. Garnish with the cilantro, lemon slices, and salt and black pepper to taste and serve.

Yield: Serves 4

CHEF'S NOTE If you like you, can use corn tortillas and the dinner will be gluten-free as well as delicious. You can also top the tacos with your favorite red or green salsa.

THREE-BEAN CHILI

No meat and yet this chili is still rich and hearty. The idea of adding the instant coffee for richness came to me in a moment of culinary risk-taking, but it turned out okay. It was delicious, in fact. Just a teaspoon gives the dish another layer of depth.

2 tablespoons (28 ml) Canna-Oil (page 18), made with olive oil

1 medium yellow onion, chopped

2 cloves of garlic, minced

1 red bell pepper, chopped

1 orange bell pepper, chopped

1 can (15 ounces, or 425 g) diced tomatoes

3 cans (15 ounces, or 425 g, each) beans, including kidney, cannellini, and great northern, rinsed and drained

2 tablespoons (32 g) tomato paste

1 teaspoon chopped fresh rosemary

1 teaspoon instant coffee powder

1 cup (200 g) pita chips, toasted

½ cup (58 g) shredded cheddar cheese (optional)

1 jalapeño chile, seeded and chopped (optional)

1 bunch of chives, chopped (optional)

1. In a medium sauté pan over medium-low heat, heat the Canna-Oil. Sauté the onion for 5 to 7 minutes until softened and translucent and then add the garlic and sauté for 2 to 3 minutes.

2. Add the bell peppers, diced tomatoes, beans, tomato paste, rosemary, and instant coffee.

3. Simmer the chili for 30 minutes until thickened to the desired consistency.

4. Serve the chili with the toasted pita chips. Top individual servings with the cheddar cheese, jalapeño, and chives, if using. Store leftovers in an airtight container in the refrigerator for up to 5 days.

Yield: Serves 6

CHEF'S NOTE If you have leftover chili, put it in a ramekin or small baking dish, top with cornbread batter, and bake.

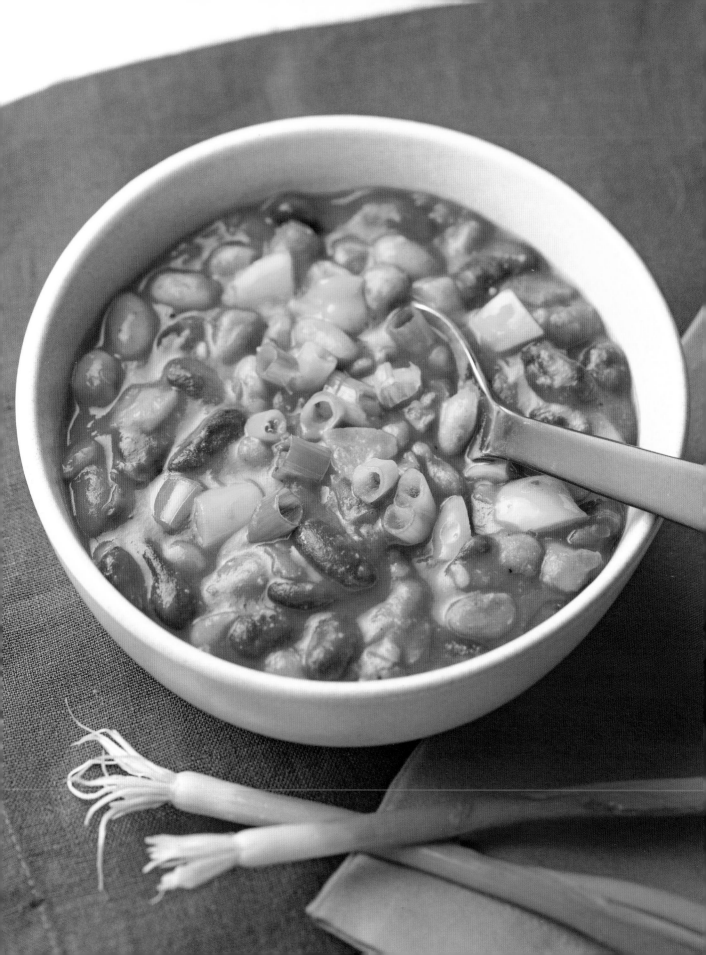

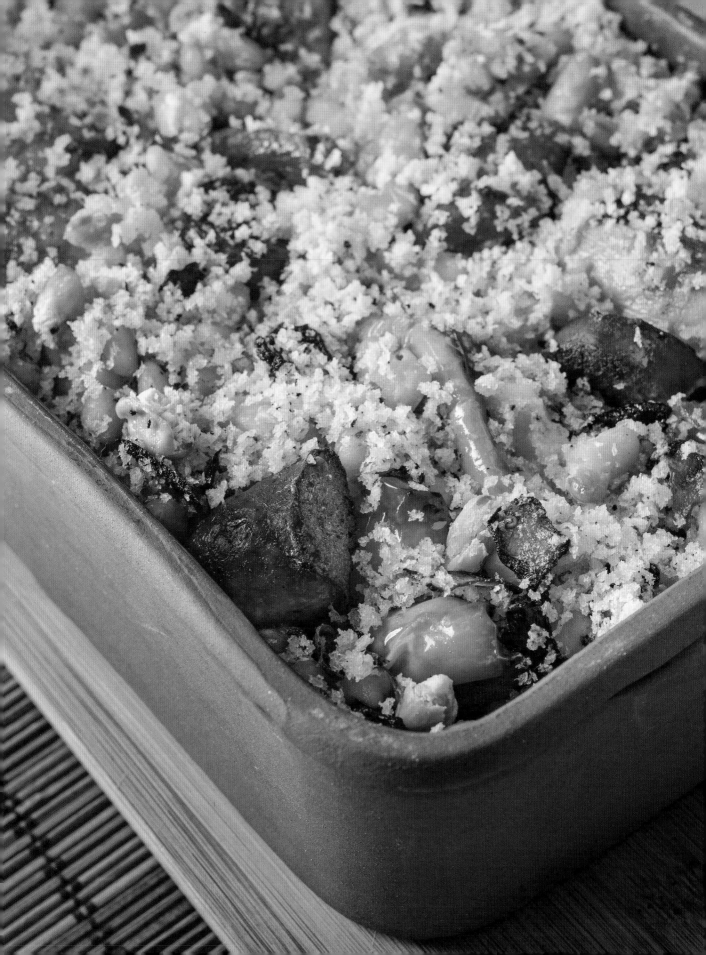

QUICK CASSOULET

Since I don't have the time to spend making a traditional cassoulet more than once every few years, I figure you might not either. This version is quick, cuts some corners, changes some ingredients, adds cannabis, and tastes great. Company always loves this dish.

2   **tablespoons (28 ml) olive oil**

2   **tablespoons (28 ml) Canna-Oil (page 18), made with olive oil**

3   **boneless, skinless chicken breasts (18 ounces, or 500 g)**

1   **yellow onion, chopped**

1   **orange bell pepper, seeded and chopped**

1   **red bell pepper, seeded and chopped**

2   **cloves of garlic, chopped**

3   **cans (15 ounces, or 425 g, each) cannellini beans, rinsed and drained**

4   **strips of bacon, cooked and chopped**

2   **kielbasa sausages (6 ounces, or 170 g), cooked and sliced into large chunks**

1   **cup (60 g) panko bread crumbs**

2   **tablespoons (8 g) chopped fresh Italian parsley**

1. Preheat the oven to 340°F (170°C, or gas mark 3).

2. In a large sauté pan over medium-high heat, heat both of the oils. Sauté the chicken breasts in the oil until golden brown on both sides, about 7 to 9 minutes. Remove and cut the chicken into large chunks.

3. In the same skillet, sauté the onion, bell peppers, and garlic over medium heat for 8 to 10 minutes until tender.

4. In a 3-quart (2.8 L) casserole dish, combine the chicken with the vegetables, beans, bacon, and kielbasa.

5. In a small bowl, combine the panko bread crumbs with the parsley. Top the casserole with the bread crumb mixture.

6. Bake the cassoulet for 35 to 40 minutes until it's bubbling and the crumb topping is turning a dark golden brown. Store leftovers in an airtight container in the refrigerator for up to 5 days.

Yield: Serves 6

CHEF'S NOTE   Pretty much a cool weather dish because of its heartiness, cassoulet is one of France's best-loved comfort foods. I have, on a couple of occasions, made this with the addition of roasted duck meat from a leftover Chinese meal.

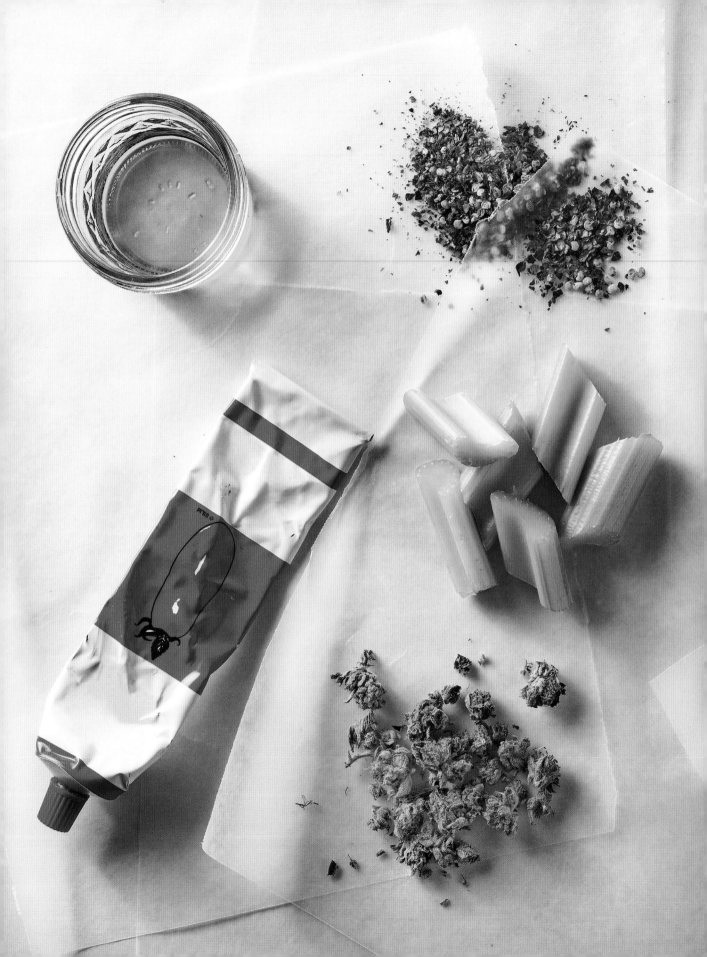

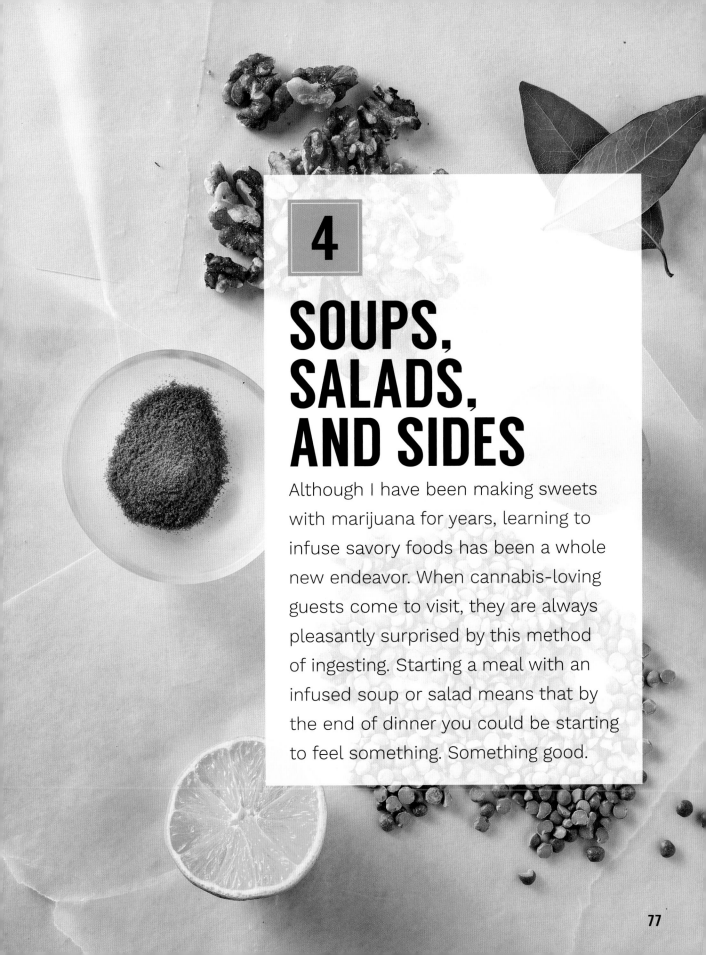

4

SOUPS, SALADS, AND SIDES

Although I have been making sweets with marijuana for years, learning to infuse savory foods has been a whole new endeavor. When cannabis-loving guests come to visit, they are always pleasantly surprised by this method of ingesting. Starting a meal with an infused soup or salad means that by the end of dinner you could be starting to feel something. Something good.

PEA SOUP WITH HAM

If this pea soup gets too thick for your tastes by the end of its cooking time, try adding a bit of broth or water to thin it out. This soup keeps for a week in the fridge and freezes beautifully.

½ pound (225 g) dried green or yellow split peas, soaked overnight in enough water to cover

4 teaspoons (20 ml) Canna-Oil (page 18), made with olive oil

½ cup (80 g) chopped yellow onion

¼ cup (25 g) chopped celery

¼ cup (33 g) finely chopped carrots

2 cloves of garlic, minced

1 ham hock, scored

2 tablespoons (8 g) chopped fresh dill

1 bay leaf

1 teaspoon salt

½ teaspoon black pepper

6 cups (1.4 L) water or vegetable or chicken broth

1. Drain the soaked peas and set aside in a medium bowl.

2. In a large soup pot, heat the Canna-Oil over medium heat. Sauté the onion, celery, carrots, and garlic for 2 to 3 minutes until they just start to soften a bit. Add the peas and the ham hock to the pot and sauté for 4 to 5 minutes. Add the dill, bay leaf, salt, and black pepper along with the water or broth.

3. Cook the soup at a low simmer for about 1 hour until it thickens to the desired consistency.

4. Remove the bay leaf and the ham hock. When the ham hock is cool enough to handle, remove the meat and add the meat back to the pot. Taste and adjust the seasoning with salt and black pepper and serve. Store leftovers in an airtight container in the refrigerator for up to 1 week or freeze for up to 3 months.

Yield: Serves 4

CHEF'S NOTE

Some people like to add sliced kielbasa or even hot dogs to their pea soup. Either is a good choice. Some folks like to make pea soup with flanken, a cut of beef that is also called short ribs. This is also a good choice! Use what you have or what sounds good to you.

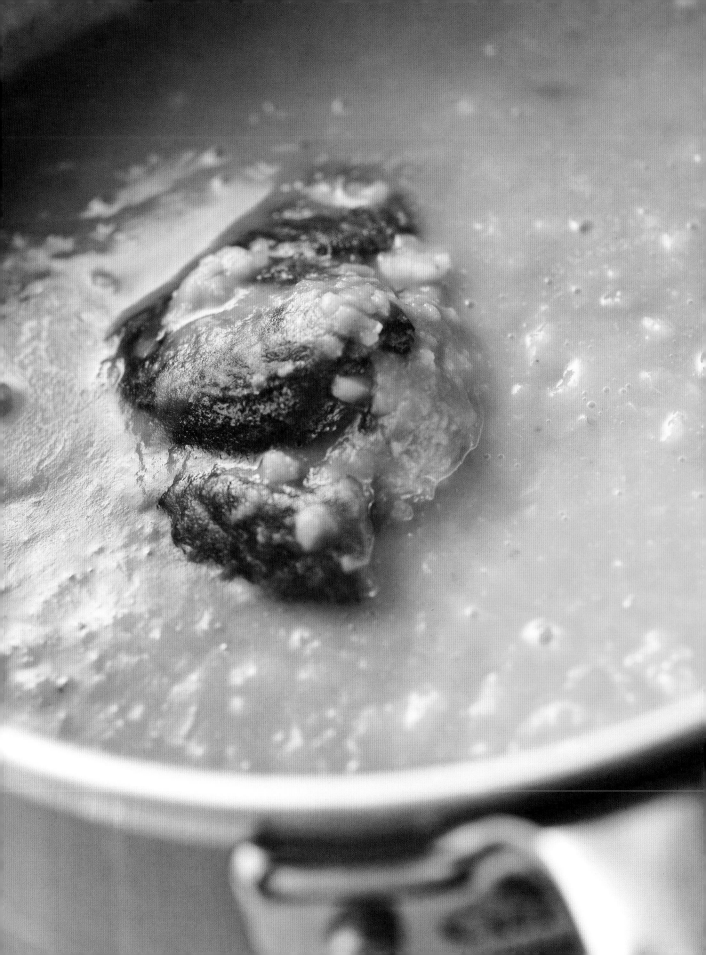

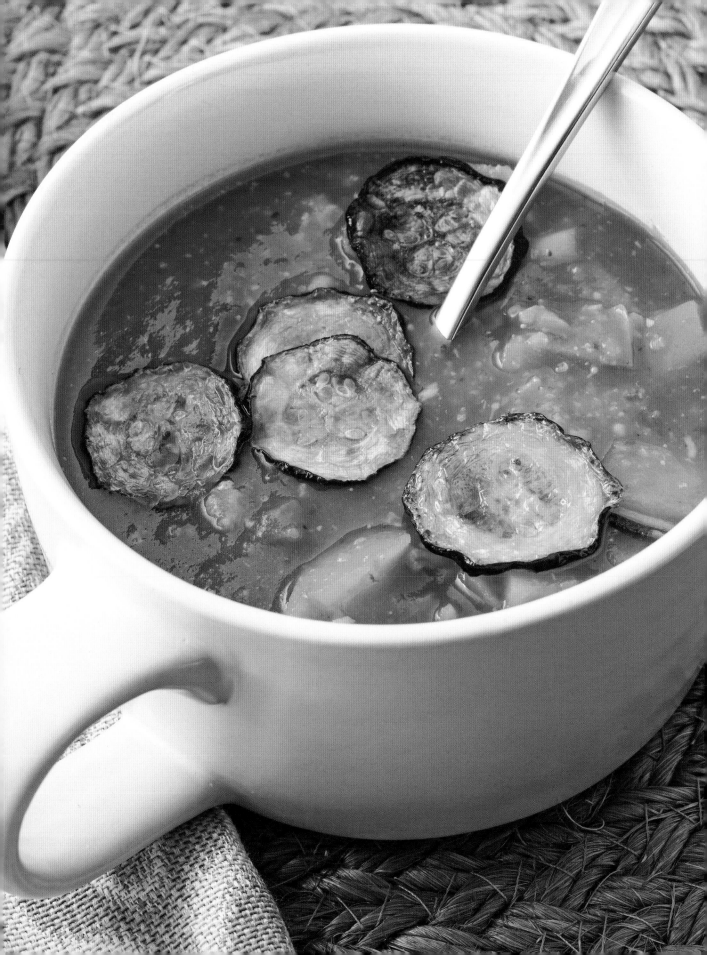

TOMATO-VEGETABLE SOUP WITH ZUCCHINI CRISPS

• Vegan

Though this soup has a lot of ingredients, it is quite simple to make. It keeps for a week and even gets better with age. But don't we all.

2 tablespoons (28 ml) Canna-Oil (page 18), made with olive oil

2 cups (260 g) chopped carrots

2 cups (240 g) chopped zucchini

12 slices of zucchini (about ¼ inch, or 6 mm, thick)

1½ cups (240 g) chopped yellow onion

1 can (14 ounces, or 390 g) fire-roasted diced tomatoes

2 cups (490 g) canned tomato sauce

2 tablespoons (32 g) tomato paste

4 cups (946 ml) water

1 teaspoon crushed red pepper

1 teaspoon salt

½ teaspoon black pepper

1 cup (150 g) fresh or (130 g) frozen green peas

1 tablespoon (15 ml) canola oil

1. In a large soup pot, heat the Canna-Oil over medium-low heat. Add the carrots, chopped zucchini, and onion and sauté for 7 to 9 minutes until the vegetables soften.

2. Add the diced tomatoes, tomato sauce, tomato paste, and the water. Cook for 45 minutes, stirring occasionally, until the soup thickens and the vegetables are tender.

3. Add the crushed red pepper, salt, and black pepper. Add the peas and cook for an additional 5 to 7 minutes.

4. In a small sauté pan over medium heat, heat the canola oil. Add the zucchini slices and stir till brown and crisp on both sides, about 7 to 9 minutes. Drain on paper towels.

5. Ladle the soup into bowls and top each serving with the zucchini chips. Store leftovers in an airtight container in the refrigerator for up to 5 days or the freezer for up to 6 months.

Yield: Serves 6

CHEF'S NOTE

Feel free to vary the vegetables here and use what you have in the house. You really can't go wrong. I recently made this soup with the addition of some spicy Italian sausage, and it was a big hit. Speaking of big hits, don't forget the Canna-Oil!

CREAMY CARROT AND POTATO SOUP

• Vegan • Gluten-free

Carrots and potatoes make such a great earthy flavor pairing, and the ground cumin and the caraway seeds deepen the flavor of this creamy, soothing soup. It's a perfect rainy night soup.

4	teaspoons (20 ml) Canna-Oil (page 18), made with olive oil
½	cup (80 g) chopped yellow onion
1½	cups (195 g) chopped carrots
2	russet potatoes, peeled and cut into chunks
1	teaspoon smoked paprika
1	teaspoon caraway seeds
½	teaspoon ground cumin
3	cups (700 ml) gluten-free vegetable broth, plus more if needed
	Chopped fresh chives, for garnish

1. In a medium soup pot, heat the Canna-Oil over medium heat. Add the onion and carrots and sauté for 7 to 9 minutes until softened. Add the potatoes, smoked paprika, caraway seeds, and cumin and sauté for 3 to 4 minutes.

2. Add the vegetable broth to the pot and simmer for 35 minutes until thickened. Add more broth if needed to achieve the desired consistency.

3. Puree the soup in a blender, in batches if necessary, until velvety smooth. Reheat if necessary. Garnish each serving with chives. Store leftovers in an airtight container in the refrigerator for up to 5 days or the freezer for up to 6 months.

Yield: Serves 4

CHEF'S NOTE

This soup also rocks with sweet potatoes instead of russet. When I serve that variation, I add a dollop of sour cream as garnish.

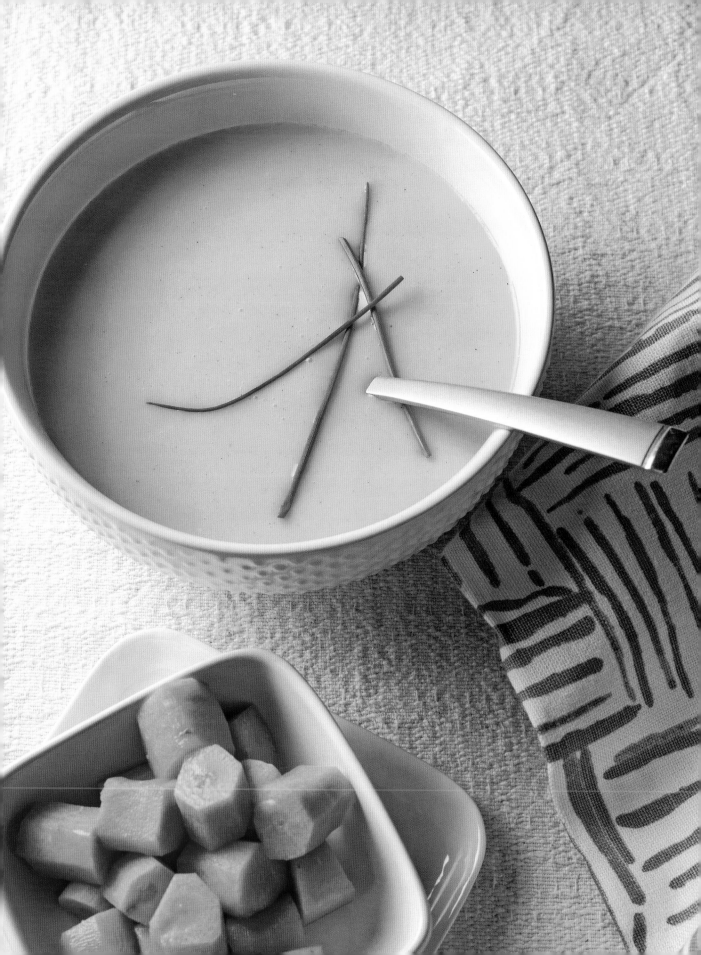

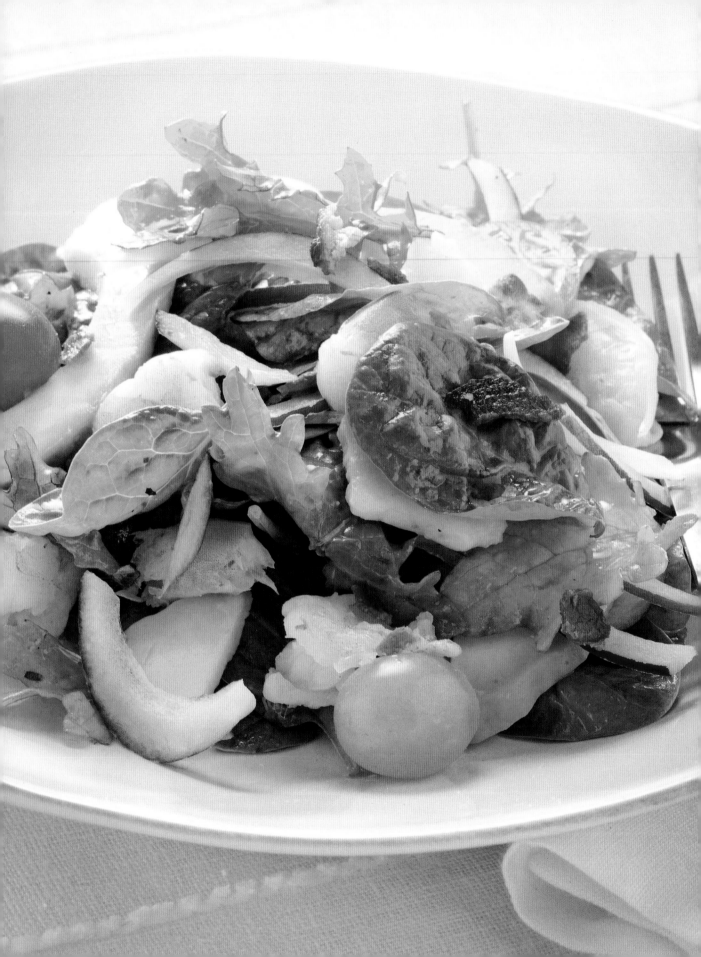

ARUGULA SALAD WITH AVOCADO AND WARM BACON VINAIGRETTE

A bacon vinaigrette is a great way to enhance a salad. The bacony deliciousness enrobes the whole thing. You can also drizzle this dressing on grilled or broiled fish or chicken.

4   strips of bacon

1   large shallot, minced

2   cloves of garlic, minced

2   tablespoons (30 g) brown sugar

6   tablespoons (90 ml) balsamic vinegar

3   tablespoons (45 ml) fresh orange juice

1   tablespoon (15 g) Dijon mustard

⅔   cup (160 ml) olive oil

4   teaspoons (20 ml) Canna-Oil (page 18), made with olive oil

8   large handfuls of mixed salad greens

20 large cooked shrimp, cut into pieces if desired

1   red onion, thinly sliced

20 grape tomatoes (cut in half if large)

1   avocado, pitted, peeled, cut into chunks or slices, and tossed with fresh lemon juice

Salt and black pepper

1. In a medium skillet over medium heat, cook the bacon until crisp. Transfer to paper towels to drain, reserving the bacon drippings in the skillet. Once cool, chop the bacon and set aside.

2. Heat the bacon drippings in the skillet over medium heat. Add the shallot and garlic and sauté for 2 to 3 minutes. Add the brown sugar and cook until dissolved, about 1 to 2 minutes.

3. Scrape the contents of the skillet into a blender. Add the balsamic vinegar, orange juice, Dijon mustard, and both of the oils. Blend well.

4. In a small bowl, toss the greens with the shrimp, red onion, tomatoes, and avocado. Add the dressing and toss again. Season with salt and black pepper to taste.

Yield: 4 (generous) servings

CHEF'S NOTE
If shrimp isn't your thing, you can substitute cooked chicken. You can also add cubes of smoked mozzarella to this salad, which gives it a very fine taste profile.

CHICKEN CAESAR SALAD

Here's one of the best salads, even for those who aren't salad lovers. The lettuce is crisp, the dressing is rich and flavorful, and the croutons are crunchy. It's easy to make your own: Just sauté leftover French bread, cut into cubes, in a bit of olive oil. They're so much better than store-bought.

3   **tablespoons (45 g) Dijon mustard**

2   **tablespoons (28 ml) fresh lemon juice**

1   **teaspoon Worcestershire sauce**

2   **cloves of garlic, smashed**

1   **anchovy fillet (optional)**

6   **tablespoons (90 ml) olive oil**

4   **teaspoons (20 ml) Canna-Oil (page 18), made with olive oil**

¼   **cup (25 g) grated Parmesan cheese**

    Salt and black pepper

2   **romaine lettuce hearts, chopped**

1   **cup (140 g) chopped or shredded cooked chicken**

2   **cups (60 g) croutons**

    Shredded Parmesan cheese, for garnish

1. In the bowl of a food processor, puree the Dijon mustard, lemon juice, Worcestershire sauce, garlic, and anchovy, if using. With the machine running, drizzle both of the oils into the bowl of the processor. Transfer the dressing to a jar and stir in the Parmesan cheese, along with salt and black pepper to taste.

2. Place the romaine in a serving bowl and toss with the dressing to coat. Top the salad with the chicken and croutons and serve immediately.

Yield: Serves 4

CHEF'S NOTE

If you like the taste of anchovy, add a couple more to the food processor when you start. It is a strange thing that people don't seem to have neutral feelings about it. Eating one as is may be a bit much for most people, but the flavor that anchovy adds to foods is pretty fabulous. Not too much—a little goes a long way.

Feel free to substitute shrimp or tofu for the chicken. The dressing is also great on all kinds of sandwiches.

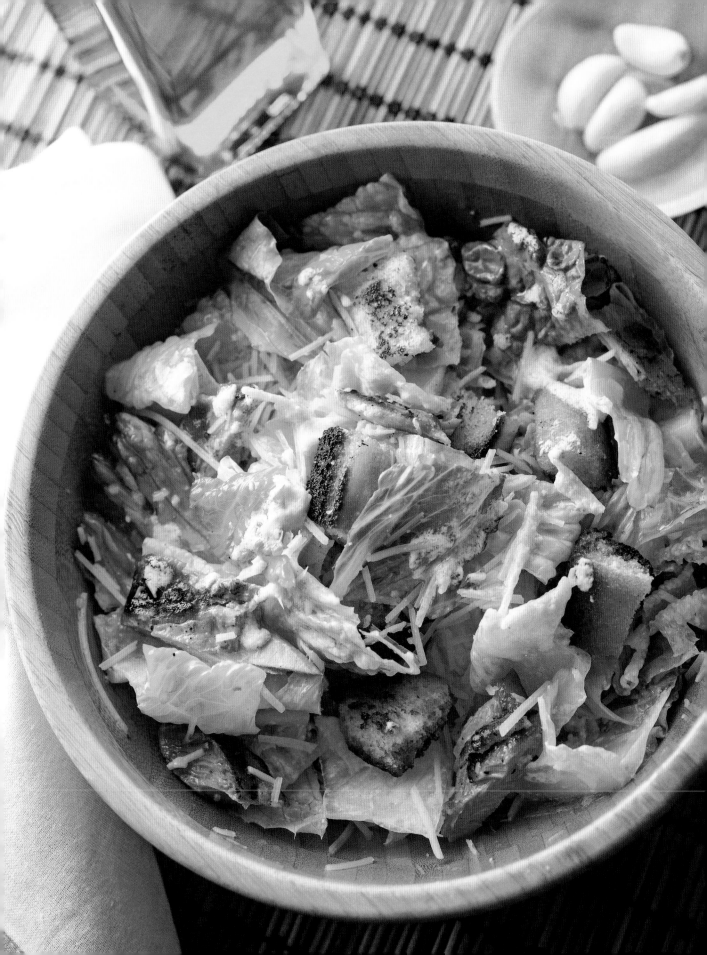

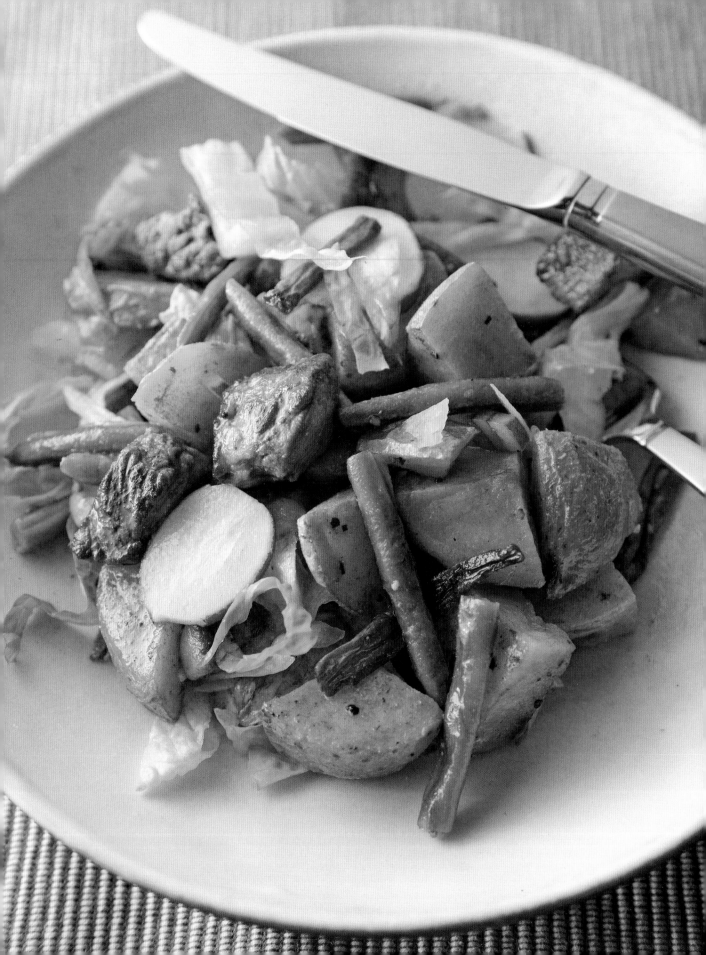

STEAK AND ROASTED POTATO SALAD

Steak and potatoes are a pretty good combo no matter how you slice it. It's worth making this salad just on the merits of the recipe, but this is also a perfect way to use up leftovers. I've given instructions for cooking the potatoes below, but you can use any leftover cooked potatoes you have in the fridge.

1 pound (455 g) skirt, hanger, or tri-tip steak

Salt and black pepper

2 pounds (900 g) small potatoes

¼ cup (60 ml) sherry vinegar

4 teaspoons (20 ml) Canna-Oil (page 18), made with olive oil

1 tablespoon (15 ml) olive oil

1 teaspoon ground cumin

1 tablespoon (15 ml) canola oil

2 scallions, cut into pieces

5 ounces (140 g) green beans, trimmed, cut into pieces, and steamed

4 cups (188 g) chopped romaine lettuce

½ cup (80 g) chopped red onion

4 radishes, thinly sliced

1. Preheat a grill for medium-high heat. Season the steak with salt and black pepper. Grill the steak until the desired degree of doneness is reached.

2. Meanwhile, to cook the potatoes, bring a pot of water to a boil. Cut the potatoes into quarters and boil until tender, about 20 minutes; drain.

3. In a medium bowl, whisk together the sherry vinegar and both of the oils. Add the cumin and salt and black pepper to taste. Set aside.

4. In a medium skillet, heat the canola oil. Add the scallions, cooked potatoes, and green beans and sauté for 4 to 5 minutes.

5. In a large bowl, combine the lettuce, steak, red onion, radishes, and cooked vegetables. Toss with the dressing and serve.

Yield: Serves 4

CHEF'S NOTE You can always change the meat or any of the vegetables to suit your tastes or what you have in the fridge. The last time I made this salad, I had some left over, which I piled onto a toasted ciabatta roll for a tasty sandwich.

WATERMELON AND FETA SALAD

• Gluten-free

I admit that I needed convincing when a friend told me about this flavor combination. But it works, especially with a hint of mint. The balance of flavors and textures is just right. It made me fall in love with watermelon again. And the seedless variety so common now is a gift from the gods.

3   cups (450 g) cubed seedless watermelon

1   cup (145 g) fresh blueberries

3   scallions, sliced

½   cup (75 g) cubed or crumbled feta cheese

2   tablespoons (28 ml) Canna-Oil (page 18), made with olive oil

1   tablespoon (15 ml) fresh lemon juice

Salt

Shredded or torn fresh mint leaves, for garnish

Lemon zest, for garnish

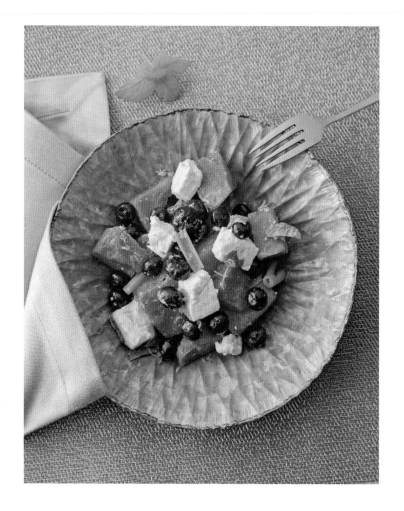

1. In a large bowl, combine the watermelon, blueberries, scallion, and feta cheese.

2. In a small bowl, whisk together the Canna-Oil with the lemon juice, salt, and mint. Pour over the fruit and toss very gently.

3. Serve very cold, garnished with the lemon zest.

Yield: Serves 6

CHEF'S NOTE Feta is a salty cheese, so adding salt may not be necessary. Taste and then decide.

CAULIFLOWER WITH CUMIN

This is just a fantastic way to prepare the under-loved cauliflower. In the past year or two, it has finally begun to get the attention it deserves. Roasting this veg is magical, and with cannabis and cumin, it becomes perfection. Plus, it looks so cool prepared this way!

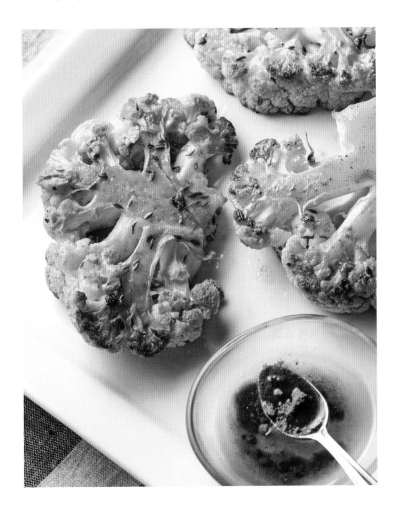

1   medium head of cauliflower, sliced into 4 slices or "steaks"

2   tablespoons (28 ml) olive oil

4   teaspoons (20 ml) Canna-Oil (page 18), made with olive oil

2   teaspoons ground cumin

1   teaspoon cumin seeds

    Salt and black pepper

1. Preheat the oven to 340°F (170°C, or gas mark 3).

2. Lay the slices of cauliflower on a rimmed baking sheet. Brush with both of the oils and sprinkle with the ground cumin, cumin seeds, and salt and black pepper to taste.

3. Roast the cauliflower until golden and tender, about 25 to 30 minutes. Serve hot.

Yield: Serves 4

CHEF'S NOTE

If you have cauliflower left over, you can turn it into a quick soup. Puree in a blender along with some hot vegetable broth and some half-and-half.

BUTTERNUT SQUASH WITH CRANBERRIES

I was originally going to develop this recipe using acorn squash. But then at a restaurant in town, I tasted a delicious butternut squash soup with a cranberry chutney. So I had to switch the squash. Both versions are good, but this is better!

2   butternut squashes

2   tablespoons (28 ml) olive oil

2   tablespoons (28 g) Canna-Butter (page 16), melted

1   tablespoon (14 g) unsalted butter, melted

¼   cup (60 ml) maple syrup

2   tablespoons (28 ml) fresh orange juice

½   cup (60 g) dried unsweetened cranberries

1. Preheat the oven to 325°F (165°C, or gas mark 3).

2. Cut the squash into 6 long sections, removing the seeds and the stringy parts (no need to peel it).

3. Toss the squash with the olive oil. Place on a rimmed baking sheet and bake for 45 minutes.

4. In a small bowl, combine the Canna-Butter, butter, maple syrup, orange juice, and cranberries. Brush the mixture onto the squash and return the baking sheet to the oven. Bake until tender, an additional 45 minutes.

Yield: Serves 6

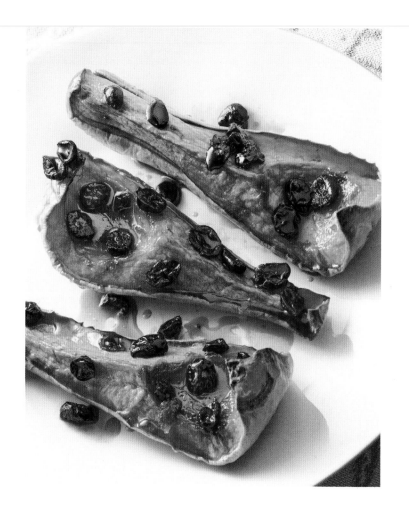

CHEF'S NOTE

For a variation, try using chopped pitted apricots and prunes instead of the cranberries.

BRUSSELS SPROUT AND PECAN STIR-FRY

Brussels sprouts have become fashionable for good reason. There are so many ways to prepare them that allow their somewhat cabbage-like flavor to shine through. Years ago, they were typically boiled beyond recognition and tasted awful. When treated properly, they're fantastic.

1 **pound (455 g) Brussels sprouts**

2 **tablespoons (28 ml) olive oil**

½ **cup (55 g) pecan pieces**

⅓ **cup (97 g) canned or jarred cooked chestnuts, chopped**

4 **teaspoons (20 ml) Canna-Oil (page 18), made with olive oil**

Juice of ½ of a lemon

Salt and black pepper

1. Shred the Brussels sprouts in a food processor. In a large skillet, heat the olive oil over medium heat. Add the Brussels sprouts and stir-fry for 2 to 3 minutes. Transfer to a bowl.

2. Add the pecans and sauté for 2 to 3 minutes. Add the chestnuts and cook for an additional 3 minutes. Add the nuts to the bowl with the Brussels sprouts.

3. Add the Canna-Oil, lemon juice, and salt and black pepper to taste and toss to combine.

Yield: Serves 4

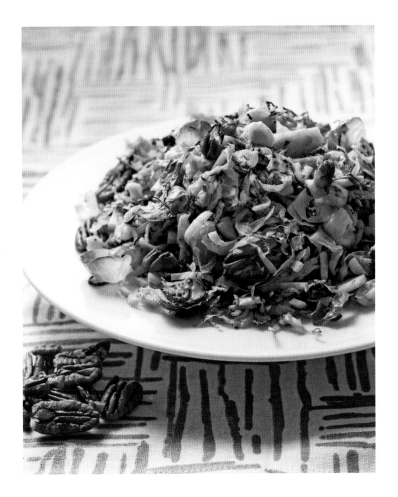

CHEF'S NOTE

This refreshing salad can be served hot or at room temperature. Add some cooked bacon and chicken for a lovely one-bowl meal.

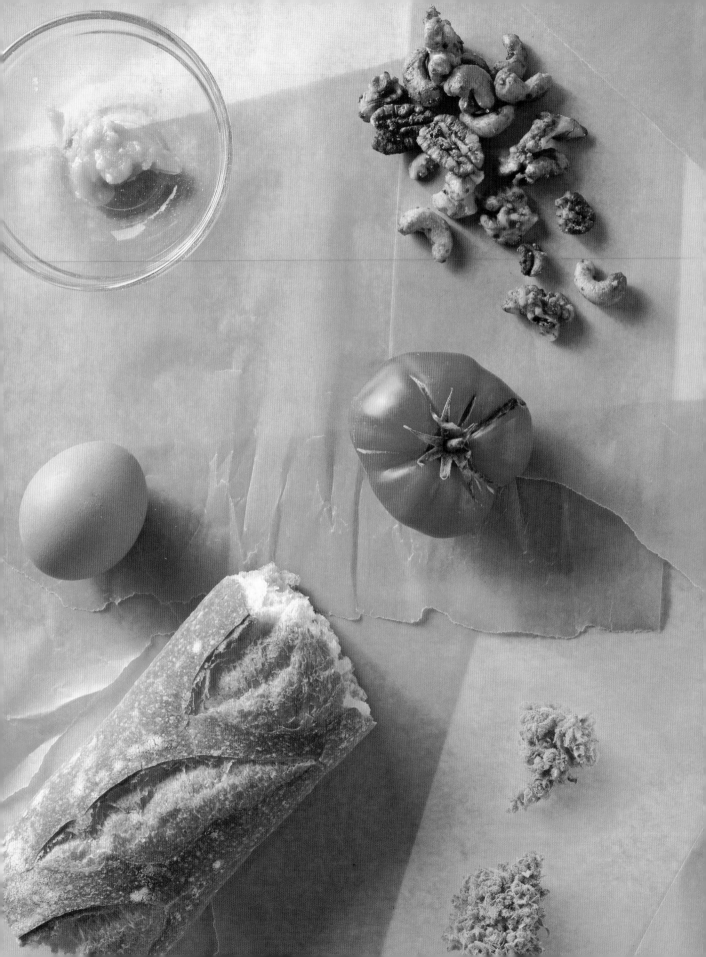

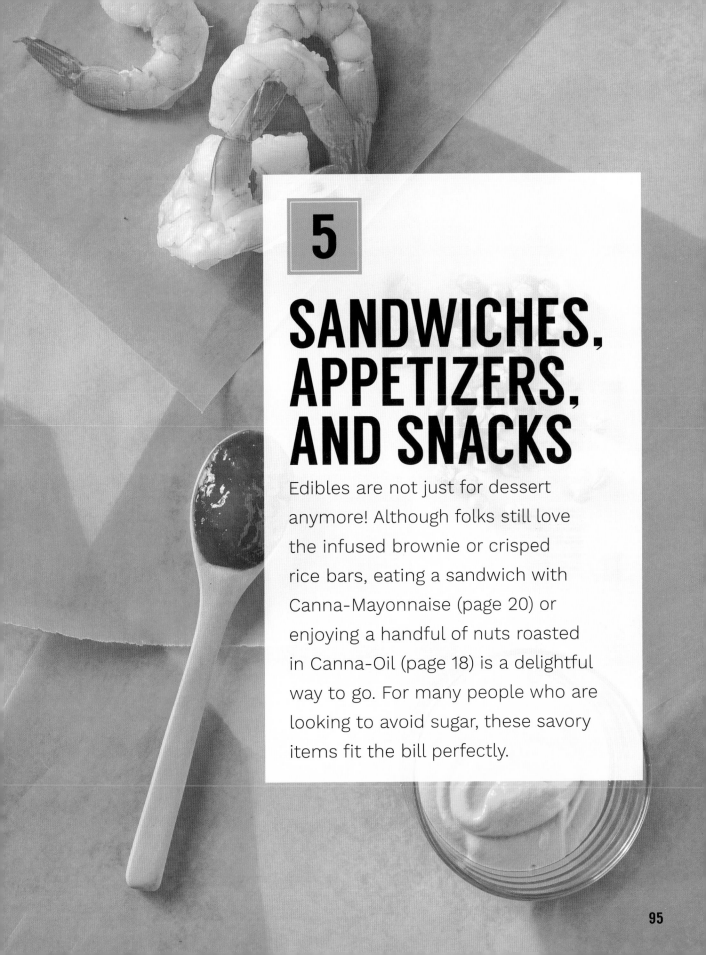

5

SANDWICHES, APPETIZERS, AND SNACKS

Edibles are not just for dessert anymore! Although folks still love the infused brownie or crisped rice bars, eating a sandwich with Canna-Mayonnaise (page 20) or enjoying a handful of nuts roasted in Canna-Oil (page 18) is a delightful way to go. For many people who are looking to avoid sugar, these savory items fit the bill perfectly.

GRILLED THREE-CHEESE SANDWICHES

There are so many cheeses to consider when attempting to make the world's greatest grilled cheese sandwich. Is there a perfect combination? I think not. Some cheeses can be ruled out due to their texture, while others can be set aside because the flavor is way too strong. That said, there is really no right or wrong choice here. It's subjective. Many think American cheese is a must, while others scoff at that plebian choice. The answer is go with what you like. Why not?

4 slices of good-quality white bread

2 teaspoons Canna-Butter (page 16), softened

2 teaspoons Dijon mustard

2 slices of cheddar cheese

2 slices of Gruyère cheese

2 slices of Muenster cheese

Pinch of salt

4 tablespoons (55 g) unsalted butter

1. Place 2 bread slices on your work surface. Spread each slice with 1 teaspoon of the Canna-Butter and 1 teaspoon of the Dijon mustard. Place the cheese slices on the bread. Sprinkle with salt. Place a top slice of bread on both sandwiches.

2. In a medium skillet, heat the butter over medium heat. When it foams, turn the heat down to medium-low and place the sandwiches in the pan. Cook on one side until golden brown and then flip the sandwiches and continue cooking until the other side is browned and the cheese is melted. Serve immediately.

Yield: Serves 2

CHEF'S NOTE

The trick is to have the cheese melted and the bread a beautiful golden color. I like to use sliced cheese, but shredded works well, though it's just a bit messier.

There are so many magnificent additions to this sandwich, including but not limited to ham, roast beef, avocado, tomato, pickles, greens. . . .

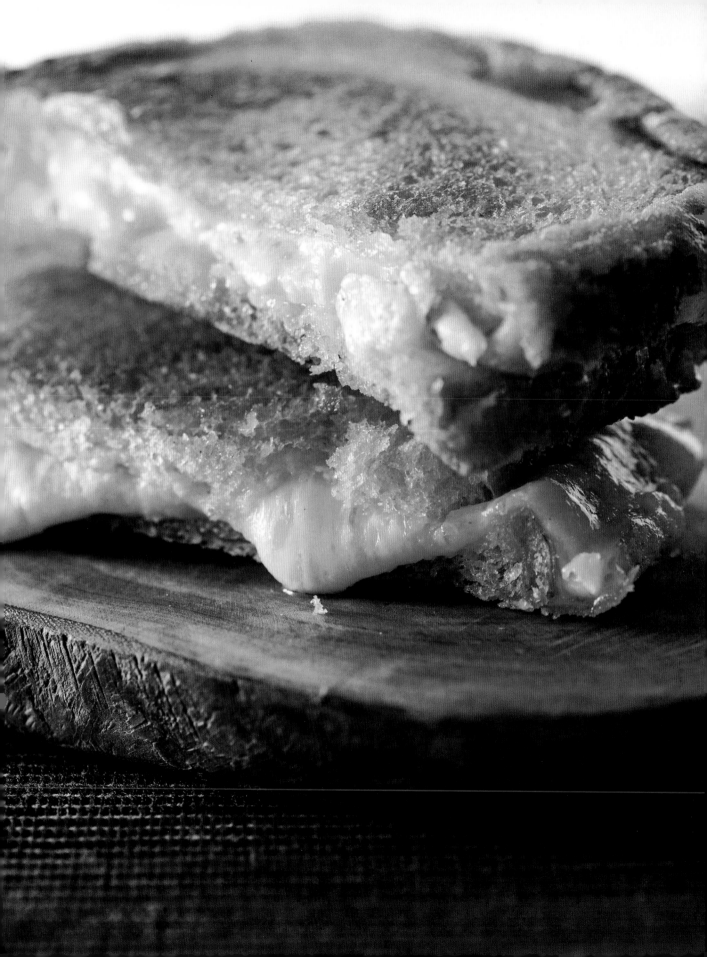

PB & J

For a change of pace, this sandwich is served open-face. Yes, you probably should use a knife and fork, but trust me—the results are extremely pleasant. The creamy peanut butter, sweet jelly, flavorful ripe banana, and a sprinkling of chopped nuts makes this worth the cutlery. Toasting the bread is optional; enjoying is not!

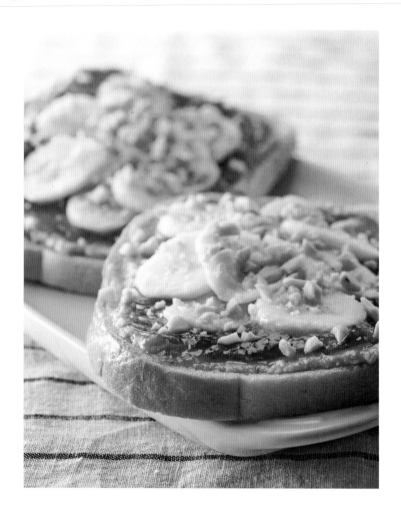

2   **slices of white bread**

6   **tablespoons (96 g) peanut butter (smooth, chunky, or a combo)**

2   **teaspoons Canna-Oil (page 18), made with coconut oil**

½   **teaspoon honey**

    Pinch of ground cinnamon

6   **tablespoons (120 g) jam, jelly, or preserves of your choice**

1   **small banana, sliced**

    Chopped roasted salted peanuts, for topping

1. Toast the bread, if you like. Place the bread on your work surface.

2. In a small bowl, combine the peanut butter with the Canna-Oil, honey, and cinnamon and spread evenly on the bread slices. Spread the jam on top of the peanut butter mixture. Divide the banana slices between the 2 slices of bread. Top with the chopped peanuts and serve.

Yield: Serves 2

BLT SANDWICHES

One of the best-loved American sandwiches, this is also perhaps the most seasonal. Without a ripe tomato, don't bother. The balance of flavors is also critical, so buy the best bacon, bread, and lettuce you can. You won't be sorry.

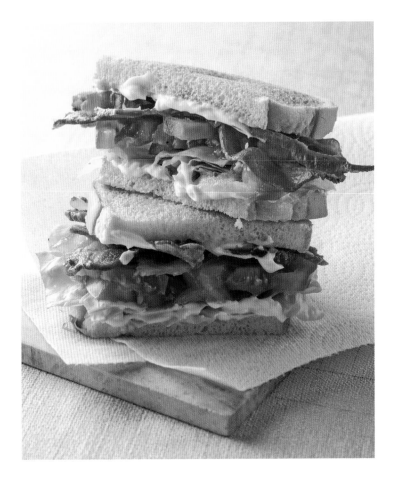

4   **slices of white bread**

4   **teaspoons (19 g) mayonnaise**

2   **teaspoons Canna-Oil (page 18), made with olive oil**

    Boston lettuce leaves

1   **ripe but firm tomato, sliced**

8   **strips of best-quality bacon, cooked to your liking**

1. Toast the bread. Place the bread slices on your work surface.

2. In a small bowl, combine the mayonnaise with the Canna-Oil. Spread on 2 of the bread slices. Top the mayonnaise with lettuce leaves. Place the tomato slices on the lettuce. Place the bacon on the lettuce and top with the remaining bread.

Yield: Serves 2

CHEF'S NOTE   You can add turkey, avocado, or even grilled shrimp to this sandwich. Once, years ago, I had a BLT with lobster, which was spectacular. However, with good-quality bacon and a ripe, juicy tomato, you truly need nothing else—besides mayo, lettuce, and bread, of course.

SHRIMP ROLLS

I can't stop making this sandwich. Seafood rolls are more traditionally made with lobster, but this shrimp roll is beyond fabulous. The fresh dill is a must, and use the freshest shrimp you can find. Some toast the bun, others don't. You can purchase cooked shrimp for the greatest convenience, or buy uncooked medium shrimp and steam them.

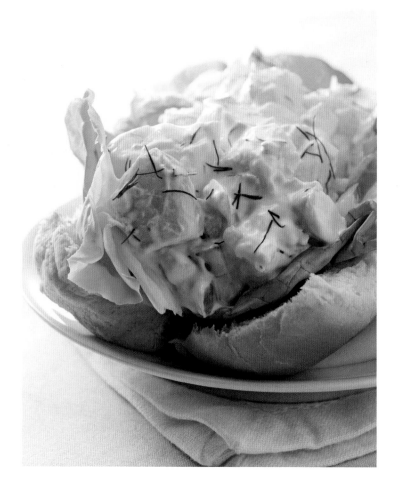

2	split-top hot dog rolls
¼	cup (60 g) mayonnaise
2	teaspoons Canna-Oil (page 18), made with olive oil
2	tablespoons (20 g) chopped red onion
1	teaspoon chopped fresh dill
2	teaspoons fresh lemon juice
¾	pound (340 g) cooked shrimp, cut into chunks
	Salt and black pepper
4	large lettuce leaves

1. Toast the rolls. Place the rolls on your work surface.

2. In a small bowl, combine the mayonnaise, Canna-Oil, red onion, dill, and lemon juice. Mix well. Add the shrimp and season with salt and black pepper to taste.

3. Line the rolls with lettuce and nestle the shrimp mixture inside. Serve immediately.

Yield: Serves 2

CHEF'S NOTE If you prefer to add fresh cilantro or parsley rather than dill, be my guest. Scallion works well as an addition, and if someone hands you a lobster, go for it.

STEAK SANDWICHES

This open-face steak sandwich is my favorite. The combination of flavors satisfies every steak-related craving. And it's a great way to use steak leftovers. Try to find a good-quality baguette and toast it lightly for sandwich perfection.

½ **pound (225 g) skirt or tri-tip steak**

Salt and black pepper

4 **pieces baguette (6 inches, or 15 cm, each)**

2 **tablespoons (28 g) mayonnaise**

2 **teaspoons Canna-Oil (page 18), made with olive oil**

1 **teaspoon prepared horseradish**

1 **clove of garlic, minced**

¼ **teaspoon crushed red pepper**

½ **of a red bell pepper, seeded and thinly sliced**

1 **small red onion, sliced**

Greens of your choice (optional)

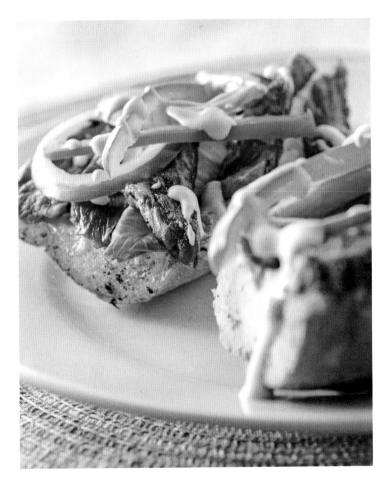

1. Preheat a grill for medium-high heat. Season the steak with salt and black pepper and grill the steak to your desired degree of doneness (4 to 5 minutes per side for medium-rare).

2. Toast the baguette pieces. Place the slices on your work surface.

3. In a small bowl, using a fork, whisk together the mayonnaise, Canna-Oil, horseradish, garlic, and crushed red pepper. Spread the mixture on the bread pieces.

4. Place the sliced steak on the toasted baguette. Top the steak with the bell pepper, red onion, and greens, if using. Serve immediately.

Yield: Serves 2

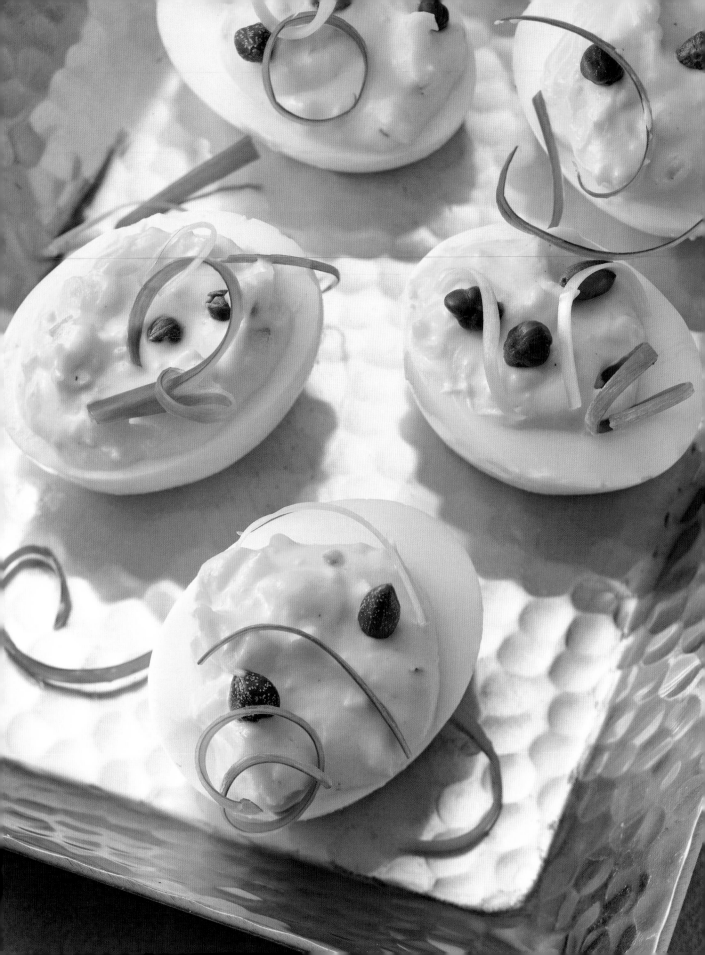

DEVILED EGGS

I never pass up an opportunity to eat deviled eggs. They seem to be trendy and on lots of menus now, I'm happy to say. Sometimes these restaurant versions are pretty complicated, but at home I tend to like them on the simple side.

4   large eggs

2   tablespoons (28 g) mayonnaise

4   teaspoons (20 ml) Canna-Oil (page 18), made with canola or olive oil

1   teaspoon finely chopped red onion

1   teaspoon capers, drained

1   teaspoon Dijon mustard

Salt and black pepper

Sliced scallion, for garnish

1. Place the eggs in a pot with cold water to cover. Bring to a boil. When the water boils, remove the pot from the heat and let the eggs sit, covered, for 18 minutes. Drain and run under cold water to stop the cooking.

2. When cool, peel the eggs. Cut the eggs in half lengthwise and remove the yolks.

3. In a small bowl, mix the mayonnaise with the Canna-Oil, egg yolks, red onion, capers, and Dijon mustard. Taste and season with salt and black pepper.

4. Spoon or pipe the filling into the egg white halves, dividing it equally. Garnish with scallions.

Yield: Serves 4

CHEF'S NOTE

A chef-friend, Kevin Gibson, tops his deviled eggs with brioche bread crumbs and then griddles them in butter. The bread crumbs form a golden brown buttery crust that is unreal. All in all, they are quite spectacular.

SPINACH, RICOTTA, AND ARTICHOKE DIP

Dips are fun, and hot dips are even more fun. This well-loved flavor combination is enhanced here with the addition of fluffy ricotta cheese and Canna-Butter. Serve this with toasted baguette slices or crackers.

1　**package (10 ounces, or 280 g) frozen chopped spinach, thawed and squeezed of excess moisture**

1　**cup (300 g) frozen artichoke hearts, thawed and chopped**

1　**package (8 ounces, or 225 g) cream cheese**

⅓　**cup (75 g) mayonnaise**

¼　**cup (45 g) ricotta cheese**

¼　**cup (60 g) sour cream**

¼　**cup (25 g) grated Romano cheese**

2　**tablespoons (28 g) Canna-Butter (page 16)**

　　Salt and black pepper

⅓　**cup (20 g) panko bread crumbs**

1　**tablespoon (14 g) unsalted butter, melted, plus 3 tablespoons (42 g), cut into cubes**

1. Preheat the oven to 340°F (170°C, or gas mark 3).

2. In the bowl of a food processor, combine the spinach, artichoke hearts, cream cheese, mayonnaise, ricotta cheese, sour cream, Romano cheese, Canna-Butter, and salt and black pepper to taste. Pulse to blend.

3. In a small bowl, combine the panko bread crumbs with the melted butter.

4. Pour the spinach mixture into an 8- or 9-inch (20 or 23 cm) baking dish and top with the bread crumbs and butter cubes. Bake for about 25 minutes until golden brown.

Yield: Serves 6

CHEF'S NOTE I have also used this dip mixture to stuff mushrooms and to spread on a turkey sandwich. It would make a delightful bruschetta topping as well.

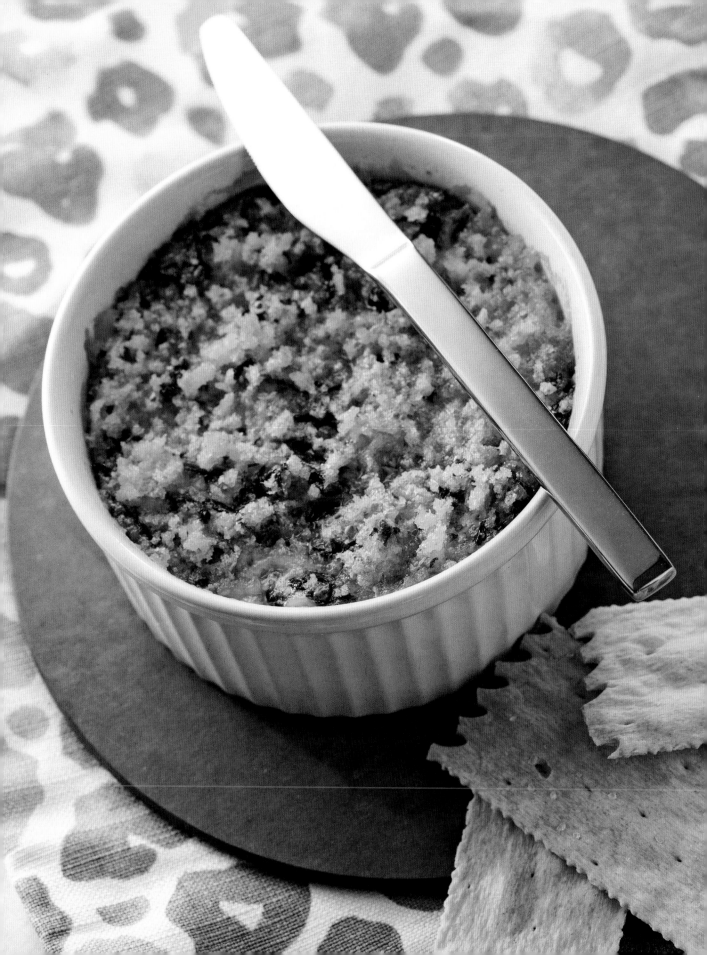

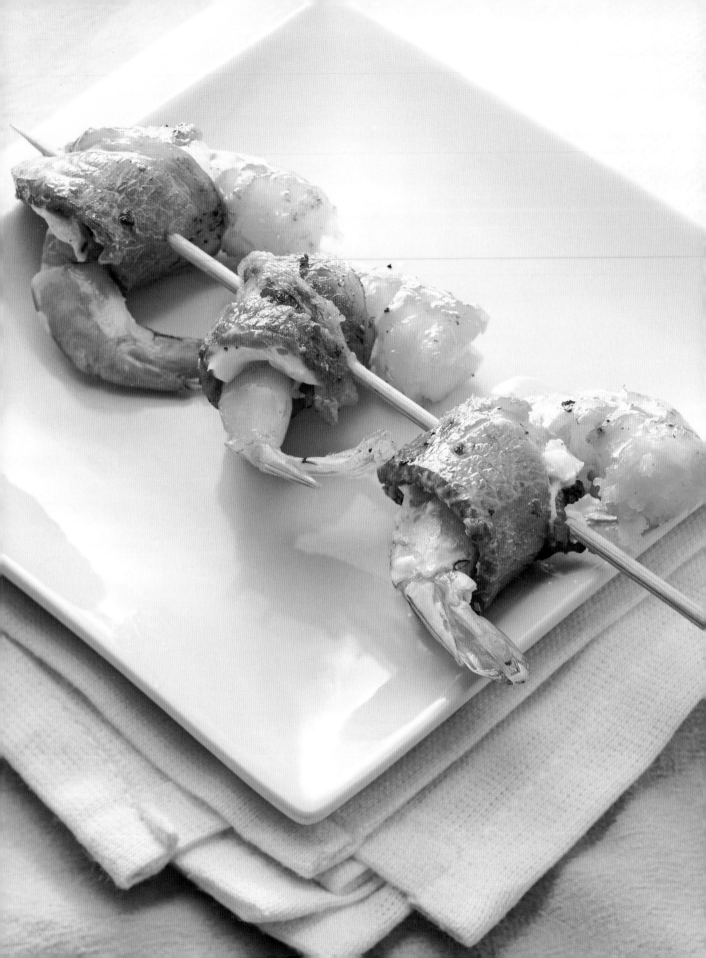

BACON-WRAPPED SHRIMP

Bacon and shrimp? Yes, please. Goat cheese, too? Amazing. And the addition of Canna-Oil takes this hors d'oeuvre or finger-food appetizer to a place that is beyond wonderful. I always try to find nitrite-free bacon. It's generally good quality and has fewer chemicals. When bacon is cooking, all but the kosher must stop and give thanks. And it tastes as good as it smells.

6   **strips of bacon, cut in half crosswise**

12   **large shrimp, peeled**

4   **teaspoons (20 ml) Canna-Oil (page 18), made with olive oil**

3   **tablespoons (28 g) goat cheese, cold**

½   **of lemon**

    Salt

1. Preheat the oven to 340°F (170°C, or gas mark 3).

2. In a medium saucepan over medium-low heat, cook the bacon about halfway. Remove from the pan and allow to cool.

3. Place the shrimp on your work surface. Brush each shrimp with the Canna-Oil.

4. Place a small piece of goat cheese on the shrimp, in the center, along with a squeeze of lemon juice and pinch of salt.

5. Wrap a piece of bacon around each shrimp, covering the cheese with the bacon. Place the wrapped shrimp on skewers, all facing in the same direction.

6. Place the bacon-wrapped shrimp, seam side down, on a rimmed baking sheet. Bake until the bacon is fully cooked and the shrimp are pink (you'll see the shrimp peeking out from the bacon), about 5 to 7 minutes.

Yield: Serves 4

CHEF'S NOTE I have also made this with blue cheese instead of goat cheese, and that's also pretty spectacular.
    The shrimp can be done on the grill as well, but be sure to soak wooden skewers in water for 30 minutes before grilling.

BAKED CAMEMBERT WITH ROSEMARY

This is a beautiful and delicious appetizer to serve with fancy crackers or breadsticks. I love the way the melted cheese spreads out as you cut into the wheel. And the Canna-Oil, walnuts, and rosemary lend a superb herbal-earthy flavor to the creamy, runny cheese.

1 **wheel (8 ounces, or 225 g) Camembert cheese**

4 **teaspoons (20 ml) Canna-Oil (page 18), made with olive oil**

2 **tablespoons (15 g) chopped walnuts**

Fresh rosemary leaves

1. Preheat the oven to 340°F (170°C, or gas mark 3).
2. Place the Camembert cheese on a rimmed baking sheet. With a knife, make small slits in the top of the cheese. Drizzle the Canna-Oil over the cheese. Top with the walnuts and rosemary. Bake for 15 to 20 minutes until the cheese is melted and runny. Serve immediately.

Yield: Serves 4

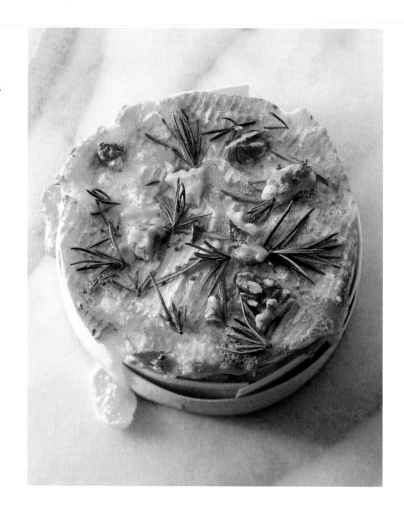

CHEF'S NOTE This also works with Brie and other similar runny cheeses enclosed in a rind. For Thanksgiving, I usually top this with fried sage leaves. It's truly an awesome appetizer.

CUCUMBER SLICES WITH SMOKED SALMON CREAM CHEESE

This refreshing snack is perfect for company. You can mix the smoked salmon into the cream cheese, but I prefer to place a little slice on top, with a squeeze of lemon juice and sometimes capers.

1 **medium cucumber, ends trimmed**

¼ **cup (60 g) cream cheese**

4 **teaspoons (19 g) Canna-Butter (page 16)**

2 **scallions, thinly sliced**

¼ **pound (115 g) smoked salmon, cut into small pieces**

½ **of a lemon (optional)**

1. Slice the cucumber and arrange on a plate.

2. In a small bowl, combine the cream cheese and Canna-Butter. Spread a bit of the cream cheese mixture on each of the cucumber slices. Sprinkle with the scallions. Top with pieces of salmon. If desired, squeeze lemon juice over the salmon.

Yield: Serves 4

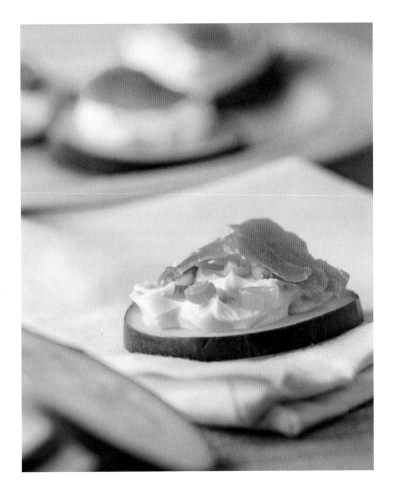

CHEF'S NOTE Taste the skin of the cucumber. If it is waxy or bitter, peel it. I like the crunch of the skin if the cucumber is homegrown.

BRUSCHETTA WITH ZUCCHINI AND RICOTTA

Zucchini is underappreciated. Here, accented with good-quality, creamy ricotta cheese and bright lemon, it is divine. Crushed red pepper gives the bruschetta a bit of spice, which works great with the mild ricotta.

8	slices of French or Italian bread
1	garlic clove, peeled and halved
2	tablespoons (28 ml) olive oil
4	teaspoons (20 ml) Canna-Oil (page 18), made with olive oil
1	small zucchini, thinly sliced
⅛	teaspoon dried oregano
⅛	teaspoon crushed red pepper
	Salt and black pepper
½	cup (125 g) ricotta cheese
1	teaspoon grated lemon zest

1. Grill or toast the bread and immediately rub the garlic clove halves over one side.

2. In a small bowl, combine both of the oils. Drizzle over the toasted bread. Set aside.

3. In a medium nonstick skillet, heat a little olive oil over medium heat. Add the zucchini and cook, stirring constantly, until the zucchini turns golden brown, about 3 to 5 minutes. Don't let it get too mushy; the zucchini should still have a little body. Remove from the heat and add the oregano, crushed red pepper, and salt and black pepper to taste.

4. Blend the ricotta cheese and lemon zest together. Divide the zucchini among the slices of bread. Top each bruschetta with 1 tablespoon (16 g) of the ricotta. Serve immediately.

Yield: Serves 4

CHEF'S NOTE

If you can grill the bread for bruschetta, that's always the best way to go. However, I don't use that method unless I am also grilling other items on the menu. If you don't want to light the grill just for bread, toasting is fine. Whichever method you use, be sure to rub the bread with the garlic clove right away. It makes for just the perfect amount of garlic every time.

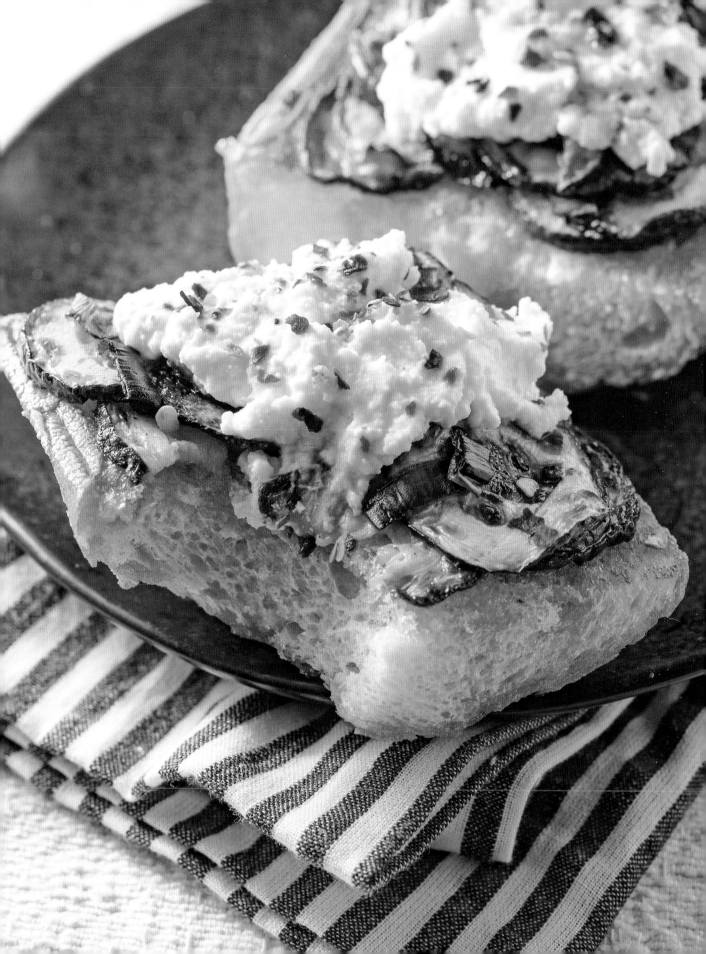

CHORIZO AND OAXACA CHEESE POTATO NACHOS

When the potatoes get crispy, they become just the perfect bed for the spicy Mexican chorizo sausage and melted Oaxaca cheese, which is sort of like a cross between Monterey Jack and mozzarella in taste and texture. The sausage is spicy, so be prepared.

2 **large russet potatoes, thinly sliced**

2 **tablespoons (28 ml) canola oil**

4 **teaspoons (20 ml) Canna-Oil (page 18), made with canola oil**

¼ **pound (115 g) bulk Mexican-style chorizo sausage**

2 **scallions, sliced**

6 **ounces (170 g) Oaxaca cheese, thinly sliced**

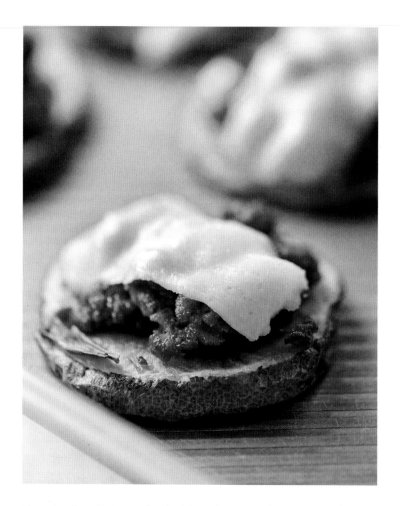

1. Preheat the oven to 325°F (165°C, or gas mark 3).

2. On a rimmed baking sheet, toss the potato slices with the canola oil. Bake for 25 to 30 minutes until crisp.

3. In a medium skillet, heat the Canna-Oil over medium-low heat. Add the chorizo and sauté for 10 minutes until fully cooked. Add the scallions and sauté for another couple of minutes.

4. Divide the chorizo evenly among the potato slices. Lay the sliced Oaxaca cheese on top of the chorizo. Return the baking sheet to the oven and bake until the cheese is melted, about 8 to 10 minutes. Serve hot.

Yield: Serves 4

MADRAS NUTS

My company, Laurie and MaryJane, won first prize at The Dope Cup
for our savory nuts. This version, with spices from India, is also
quite a crowd-pleaser.

1 cup (100 g) unsalted
pecan halves

1 cup (140 g) unsalted cashews

1 cup (100 g) unsalted
walnut halves

2 tablespoons (12 g)
curry powder

1 teaspoon ground cumin

½ teaspoon ground cardamom

Pinch of cayenne pepper

Salt

3 tablespoons (45 ml)
Canna-Oil (page 18),
made with canola oil

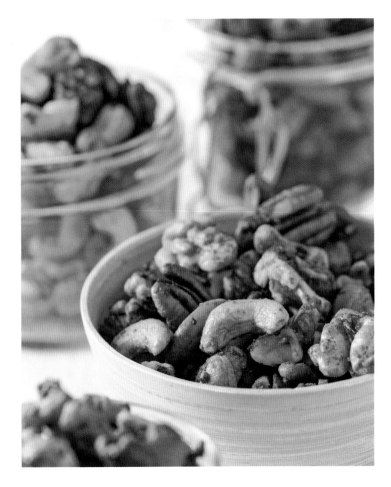

1. Preheat the oven to 300°F
(150°C, or gas mark 2).

2. On a rimmed baking sheet,
combine all of the ingredients,
mixing well to ensure even
distribution of the spices.

3. Bake for 20 to 25 minutes,
stirring occasionally, until the
nuts have darkened slightly and
are very aromatic.

4. Allow the nuts to cool completely. Store in
an airtight container.

Yield: Serves 9

CHEF'S NOTE

If you want to try a different spice flavor profile, go the Latin route and
use ½ teaspoon chili powder, ½ teaspoon ground cumin, ¼ teaspoon
ground ginger, and a pinch of cayenne pepper.

TORTILLA PIZZA

I don't know too many people who have the time to make pizza dough from scratch. There are always those prebaked pizza shells, but this recipe shows how I like to roll. Load up a tortilla with your toppings of choice and you have a pizza in just minutes!

½ pound (225 g) bulk Italian sausage

4 large flour tortillas

4 teaspoons (20 ml) Canna-Oil (page 18), made with olive oil

⅔ cup (163 ml) tomato sauce of your choice, mixed with 4 teaspoons (20 ml) Canna-Oil (page 18) made with olive oil

1 small red onion, chopped

1 cup (115 g) shredded mozzarella cheese

½ cup (40 g) shredded Parmesan cheese

1. Preheat the oven to 340°F (170°C, or gas mark 3).
2. In a medium skillet over medium heat, cook the sausage, stirring frequently. The sausage should turn brown and have no visible pink remaining.
3. Place the tortillas on a baking sheet and spread 1 teaspoon of Canna-Oil on each tortilla.

Top with the tomato sauce. Add the sausage, red onion, and mozzarella and parmesan cheese to each pizza.
4. Bake until the cheese melts and the crust turns golden brown around the edges, about 5 to 7 minutes.

Yield: Serves 4

PIZZA AND CANNABIS

If you are willing to entertain a rather loose definition of pizza, it's a great food to infuse. As a base you can use any of the following:

English muffins • Corn tortillas • Flour tortillas
Puff pastry • Pie dough • Flatbreads • Baguettes
Bagels • Pitas

The infusion materials can be Canna-Butter or any type of Canna-Oil, incorporated by either brushing the base with the infused ingredient or sautéing the toppings in the Canna-Butter or Canna-Oil. Here are a few combos to get you going:

• Corn kernels and bacon on a corn tortilla with cotija cheese
• Pesto and smoked mozzarella on flatbread
• English muffin with tomato, cheddar, and avocado
• Puff pastry with tomato, sausage, and Fontina cheese

CHEF'S NOTE Remember that pizza does not always mean red sauce. Try drizzling the tortillas with Canna-Oil and then topping them with three different cheeses or chopped sautéed vegetables and maybe an egg.

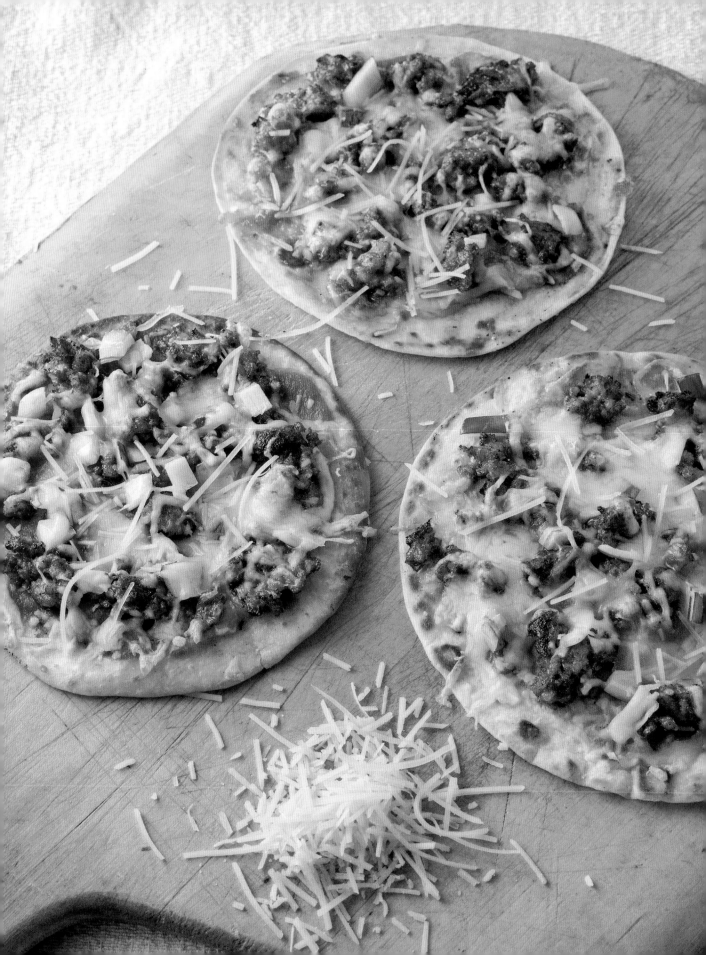

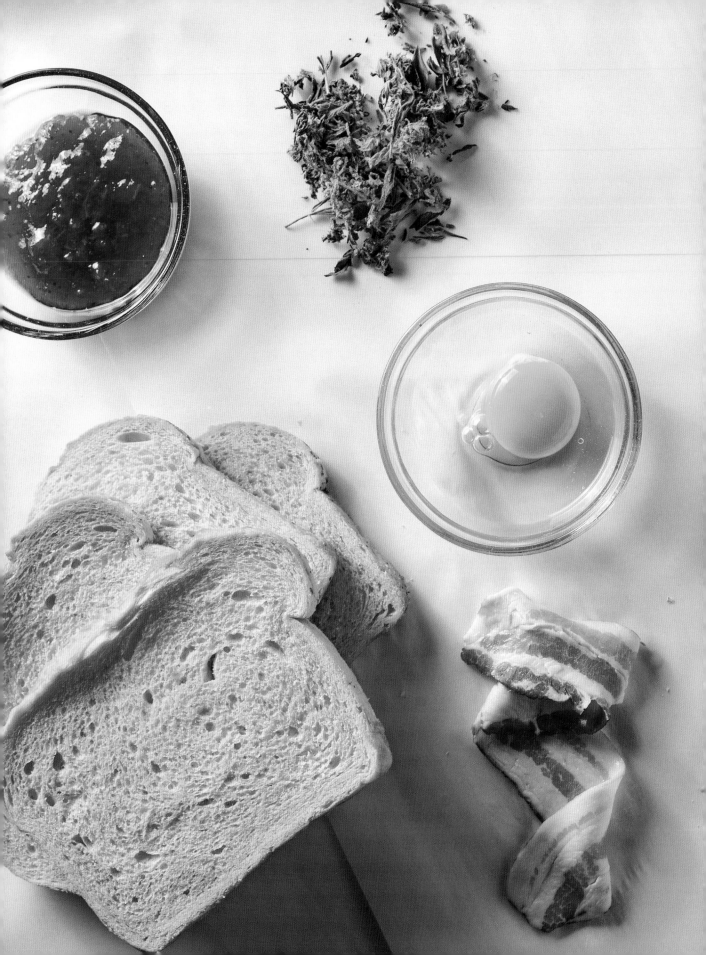

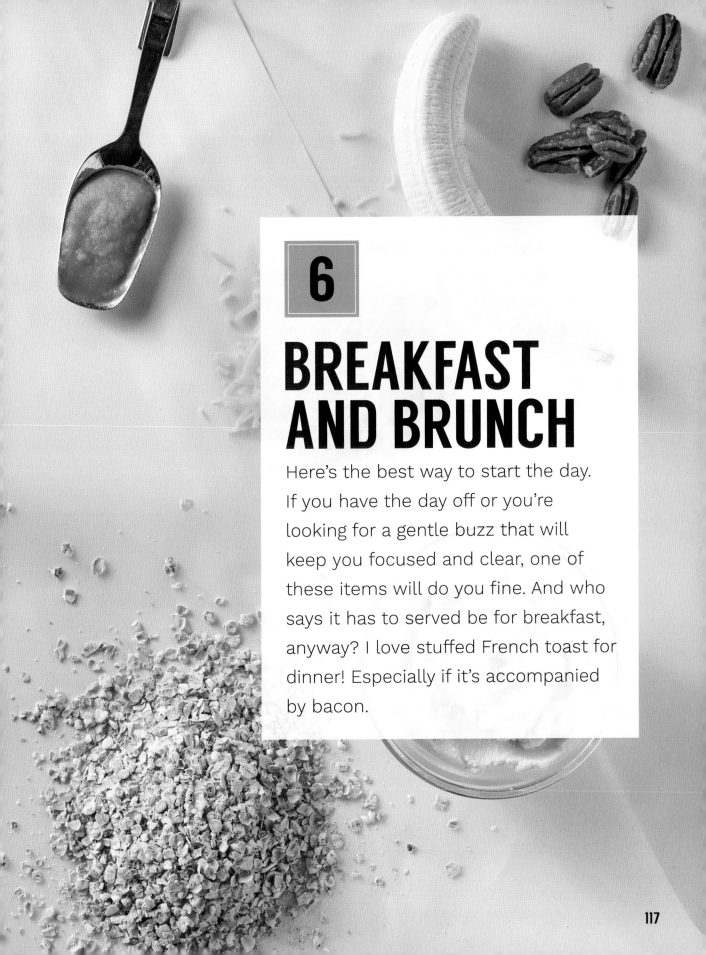

6

BREAKFAST AND BRUNCH

Here's the best way to start the day. If you have the day off or you're looking for a gentle buzz that will keep you focused and clear, one of these items will do you fine. And who says it has to served be for breakfast, anyway? I love stuffed French toast for dinner! Especially if it's accompanied by bacon.

STUFFED FRENCH TOAST

Starting your day with cannabis-infused French toast seems just too good to be true. The ricotta and the jam combine to make just the right level of creamy, tangy sweetness.

4   slices of white bread

2   teaspoons Canna-Butter (page 16), melted

¼   cup (65 g) ricotta cheese

¼   cup (80 g) jam of your choice

2   large eggs, lightly beaten

1   tablespoon (15 ml) milk

3   tablespoons (42 g) unsalted butter

     Confectioner's sugar, for garnish (optional)

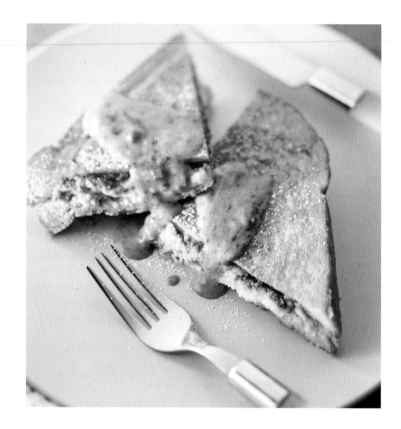

1. Brush 2 slices of the bread with the melted Canna-Butter. Layer the 2 slices with the ricotta cheese and then the jam. Top off each sandwich with a slice of bread.

2. In a wide, shallow bowl, beat the eggs and milk. Dip the sandwiches into the egg mixture.

3. In a large skillet, melt the butter over medium heat. When the butter starts to foam, add the sandwiches. Cook until golden brown, about 3 to 4 minutes, and then turn and cook on the other side until golden brown.

4. Place on serving plates, cut in half, drizzle with any remaining jam, and sprinkle with confectioner's sugar, if using.

Yield: Serves 2

CHEF'S NOTE

For picture-perfect confectioner's sugar sprinkling, use a small tea strainer or sifter. Feel free to vary the jam flavor as you like; apricot is always a good choice.

BACON AND EGG MUFFINS

This is an easy breakfast that everyone adores. It looks like it was tons of trouble to make, but it's a cinch. It's really yummy with shredded Swiss cheese as well, and you can also substitute sautéed spinach for the bacon.

4   flour tortillas
    (6 inch, or 15 cm)
4   teaspoons (19 g) Canna-
    Butter (page 16), melted
1   cup (115 g) shredded
    cheddar cheese
4   strips of bacon, cooked
    and chopped
4   large eggs, at room
    temperature
    Salt and black pepper

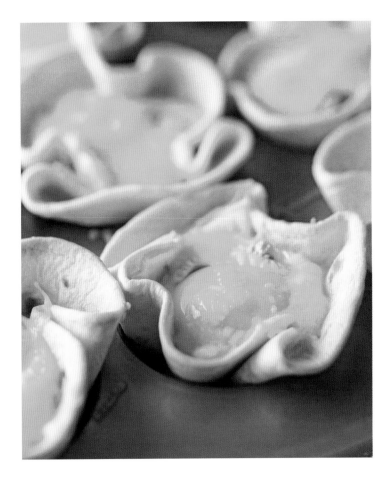

1. Preheat the oven to 340°F (170°C, or gas mark 3).

2. Press the flour tortillas into 4 cups in a standard-size muffin pan. Brush the inside of the tortilla cups with the Canna-Butter.

3. Divide ¾ cup (86 g) of the cheddar cheese among the tortilla cups. Top with the chopped bacon. Carefully break an egg into each tortilla cup. Top evenly with the remaining cheese. Sprinkle with salt and black pepper.

4. Bake until the eggs are set, about 10 minutes. Serve immediately.

Yield: Serves 4

CHEF'S NOTE

If the tortillas seem brittle, heat them in the microwave for 10 seconds to soften them. To bring the eggs to room temperature, place them in a bowl of tepid water for 20 minutes.

OATMEAL WITH THE WORKS

Try to use the best-quality oatmeal you can afford because it really does make a difference. Steel-cut oats are nice and chewy. This is such a cozy way to start the day.

3¼ cups (765 ml) water

2 cups (160 g) steel-cut oats

Pinch of salt

4 teaspoons (19 g) Canna-Butter (page 16)

1 banana, peeled and sliced

4 tablespoons (28 g) chopped pecans

4 tablespoons (30 g) chopped walnuts

2 tablespoons (20 g) dried cherries

2 tablespoons (40 g) honey

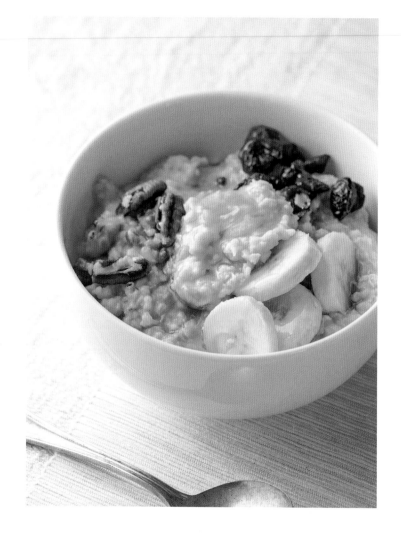

1. In a large pot, bring the water to a boil. Add the oats and salt and gently simmer for 5 minutes. Remove from the heat and let rest, covered, for 2 minutes. Stir in the Canna-Butter.

2. Divide the oatmeal among 4 bowls and evenly top with the remaining ingredients. Serve immediately.

Yield: Serves 4

CHEF'S NOTE When I have leftover oatmeal, I make pancakes. Add an egg, a few splashes of milk, a bit of baking soda, and whatever spices you like to the oatmeal. Dollop the batter onto a griddle, and you have recycled one great breakfast into another.

BREAKFAST PARFAITS

Starting the day off with this breakfast feels decadent, but it's easy to make and healthy too. It can be prepared the night before, but just be aware that the granola will get a bit soggy where it meets the yogurt. It's no biggie. You can use the infused granola on page 122 to make the parfaits, but in that case you might want to use plain coconut oil rather than the Canna-Oil.

2   teaspoons Canna-Oil (page 18), made with coconut oil

2   teaspoons honey

1   cup (125 g) granola

2   peaches, sliced

1   cup (230 g) yogurt, in your choice of flavor

1. Preheat the oven to 340°F (170°C, or gas mark 3).

2. In a medium bowl, combine the Canna-Oil and honey until blended. Add the granola and stir to coat well. Spread out on a rimmed baking sheet. Bake for 5 to 7 minutes. Allow to cool.

3. Layer ¼ cup (31 g) of the granola on the bottom of each of 2 bowls or glasses. Top with peaches. Follow with ¼ cup (60 g) of yogurt. Repeat, then top with a few more peach slices and serve.

Yield: Serves 2

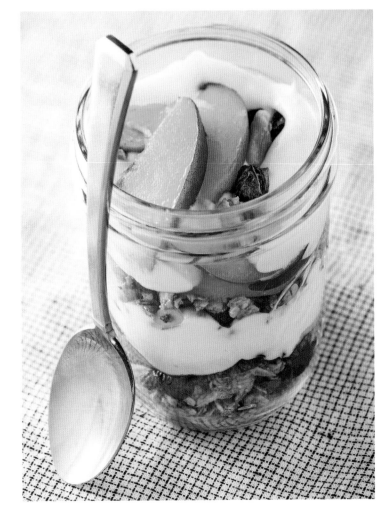

CHEF'S NOTE   This parfait tastes great with ricotta cheese or cottage cheese too, instead of yogurt. Cottage cheese is underappreciated, in my opinion, and I think it's going to make a comeback. Just wait.

GRANOLA

Homemade granola is so much better than the store-bought variety. You can keep it simple and classic or add a ton of extra ingredients. This version is so good that you'll just want to eat it plain. And it makes a nice gift as well, packaged in a pretty jar.

5 tablespoons (100 g) honey

¼ cup (60 ml) Canna-Oil (page 18), made with coconut oil, or Canna-Butter (page 16), melted

4 cups (320 g) old-fashioned rolled oats

⅓ cup (47 g) unsalted cashews, chopped

½ cup (30 g) unsweetened coconut flakes

1 teaspoon ground cinnamon

½ cup (65 g) dried apricots, chopped

¼ cup (40 g) dried cherries or (35 g) raisins (optional)

1. Preheat the oven to 300°F (150°C, or gas mark 2).
2. In a large bowl, combine the honey and Canna-Oil and stir well. Add the oats and stir again to coat all of the oats evenly. Add the cashews, coconut flakes, and cinnamon and toss to combine. Transfer to a rimmed baking sheet.
3. Bake, stirring occasionally, for about 20 minutes, and then remove from the oven and stir in the dried apricots and cherries. Return to the oven and bake, stirring occasionally, for another 15 to 20 minutes until golden brown. Let cool on the baking sheet. The mixture will be sticky at first, but once it cools it will be perfect. And it's perfectly delicious.

Yield: Serves 12

CHEF'S NOTE If you use raisins instead of cherries, you may want to add them only 5 or 10 minutes before the end of the baking time. I like when they cook and get kind of dark and chewy, but I realize that not everyone does.

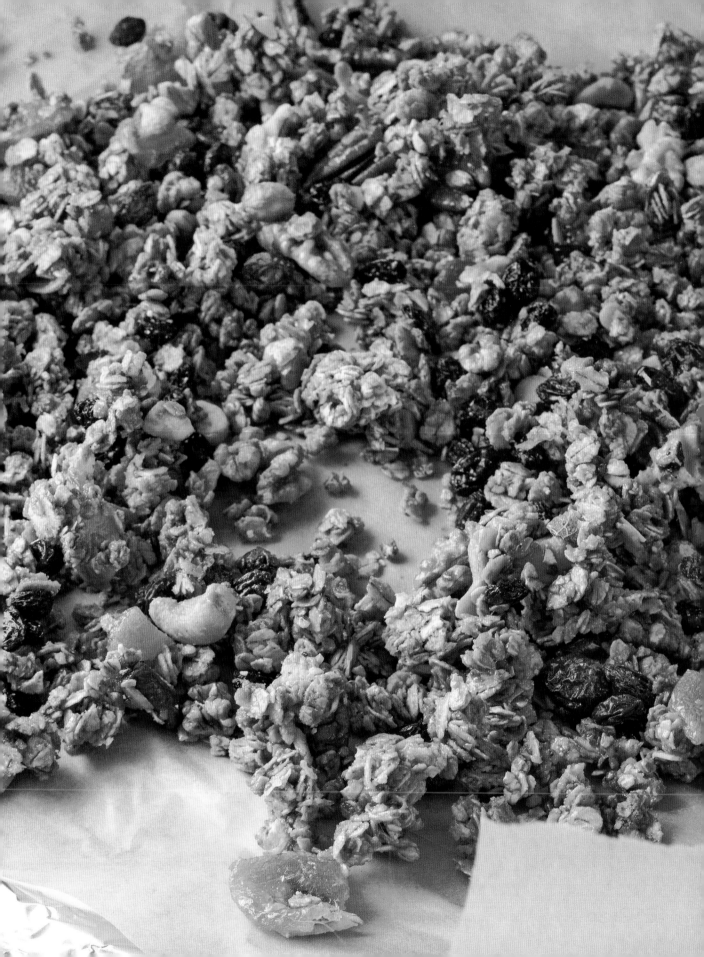

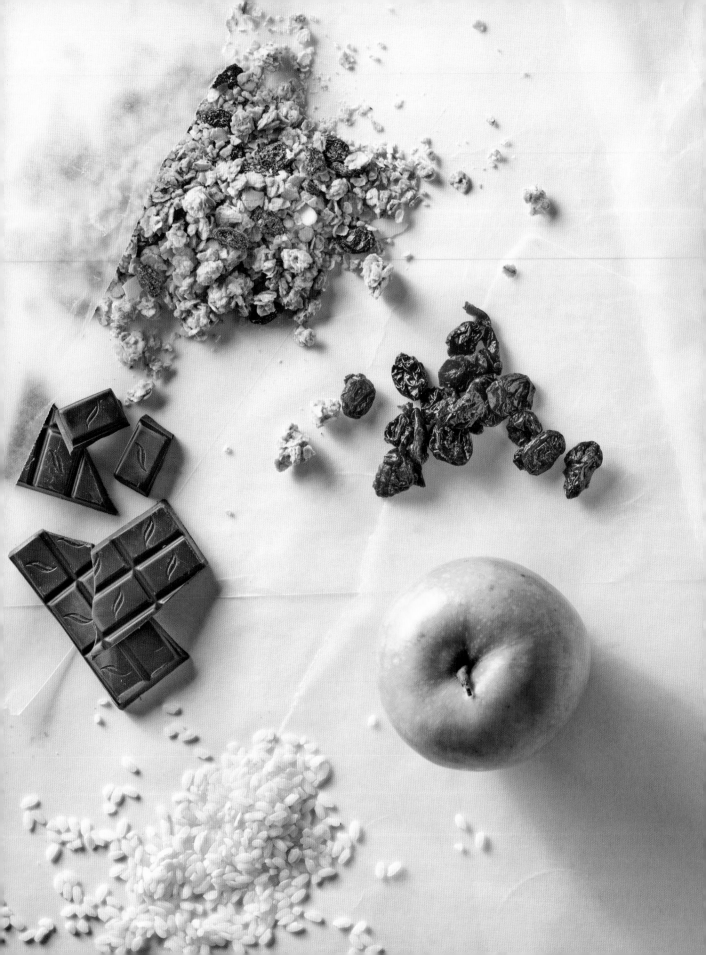

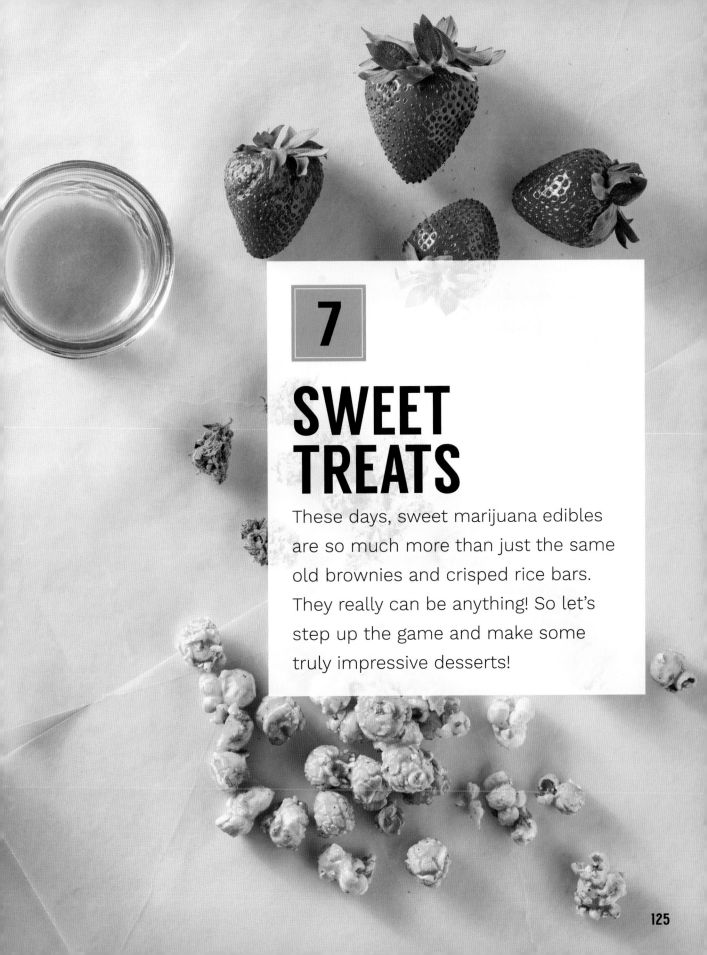

7

SWEET TREATS

These days, sweet marijuana edibles are so much more than just the same old brownies and crisped rice bars. They really can be anything! So let's step up the game and make some truly impressive desserts!

CHOCOLATE BARK WITH PECANS, COCONUT, AND APRICOTS

This is so unbelievably easy to make you could have this in the house all the time. But then it would not be special. Does it have to be special? You decide. Maybe it just has to be amazingly yummy.

½ cup (30 g) unsweetened coconut flakes

2 cups (350 g) dark chocolate chips or melts

3 tablespoons (42 g) Canna-Butter (page 16)

½ cup (55 g) chopped pecans

¼ cup (33 g) dried apricots

1. Place the coconut flakes in a small dry skillet over medium heat and toast until pale golden brown. Transfer to a bowl to prevent from getting any darker.

2. In the top of a double boiler over simmering water, melt the chocolate chips with the Canna-Butter, stirring occasionally.

3. Place a piece of parchment paper on your work surface. Pour the chocolate onto the parchment, spreading it out to about a 5 x 7-inch (13 x 18 cm) rectangle.

4. Sprinkle the chocolate with the pecans, toasted coconut flakes, and dried apricots.

5. Allow the chocolate to set at room temperature for at least 1 hour before breaking into pieces. Store in an airtight container at room temperature for up to 1 month.

Yield: Serves 9

CHEF'S NOTE

Chocolate melts take the worry out of working with chocolate because you don't have to worry about the chocolate burning or seizing. They are, however, not as good as pure chocolate because they have other ingredients added and therefore a less chocolaty flavor. This is an age-old struggle and you must decide for yourself.

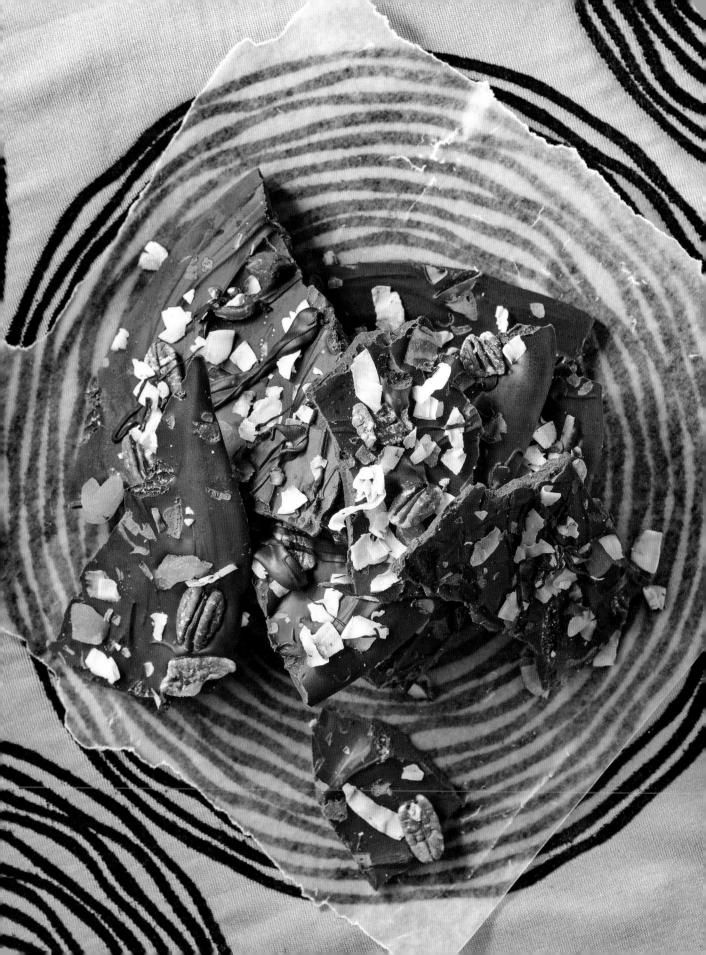

WHITE CHOCOLATE BARK WITH DRIED CHERRIES AND GRANOLA

Cannabis and white chocolate are delicious together. It seems like each ingredient just brings out the best in the other. Dried cherries and granola gild the proverbial lily. If you would like to use the infused granola on page 122, I suggest you use regular unsalted butter instead of the Canna-Butter.

2 cups (350 g) white chocolate chips or melts

3 tablespoons (42 g) Canna-Butter (page 16)

1 cup (125 g) granola

⅓ cup (53 g) dried cherries

1. In the top of a double boiler over simmering water, melt the white chocolate chips with the Canna-Butter, stirring occasionally.

2. Place a sheet of parchment paper on your work surface. Pour the white chocolate onto the parchment, spreading it out to about a 5 x 7-inch (13 x 18 cm) rectangle. Sprinkle the white chocolate with the granola and the dried cherries.

3. Allow to set for at least 1 hour before breaking into pieces. Store in an airtight container at room temperature for up to 1 month.

Yield: Serves 8

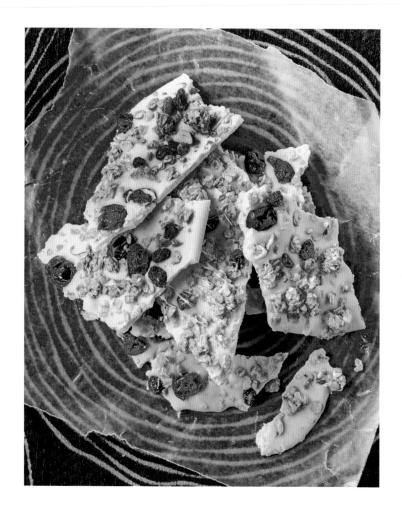

CHEF'S NOTE

Instead of cherries and granola, try crumbled graham crackers and mini marshmallows. It's hard to go wrong with that!

TRIFLE WITH BERRIES

Instead of the traditional custard, which can be time-consuming to prepare, I use Greek yogurt here, which is just as creamy, better for you, and totally delicious. If you want to prepare your trifles the day before you serve them, make them in little mason jars, store them in the refrigerator with the lids on, and then add the whipped cream right before serving—so easy, so cute, and so delicious.

1½ cups (340 g) pound or angel food cake crumbs (from a 9- or 10-inch [23 or 25.5 cm] cake)

1½ cups (approximately 220 g) fresh berries of your choice

1½ cups (345 g) vanilla Greek yogurt

2   tablespoons (28 g) Canna-Butter (page 16), melted and cooled

Whipped cream, for topping

Fresh berries, for garnish

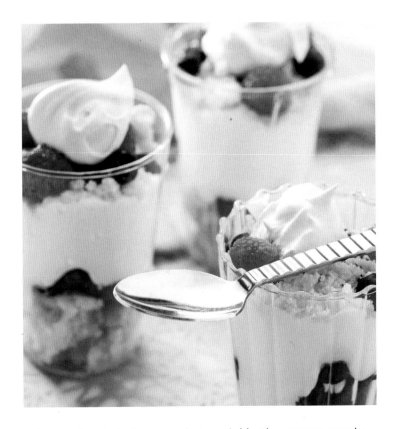

1. Set aside 3 tablespoons (45 g) of the cake crumbs for garnish. Divide the remaining cake crumbs evenly among six 8-ounce (235 ml) containers. Sprinkle the berries over the cake crumbs. In a small bowl, combine the Greek yogurt with the Canna-Butter. Distribute the yogurt mixture evenly among the containers, placing it on top of the berries.

2. Immediately before serving, sprinkle the yogurt evenly with the reserved cake crumbs, top with whipped cream, and garnish with berries.

Yield: Serves 6

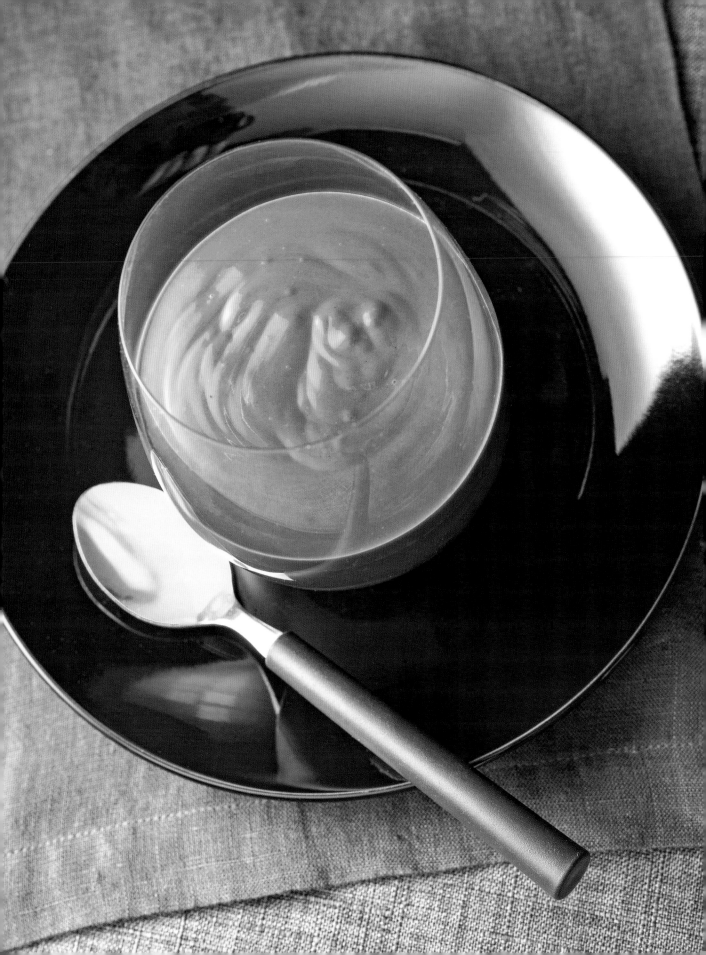

EASY CHOCOLATE PUDDING

I don't generally like to garnish this pudding. You could certainly top it with some fresh berries, some whipped cream, or even a little pool of heavy cream. But there is something about the rich, deep chocolaty flavor of this pudding that I prefer not to adulterate. I like to serve this pudding in some kind of wine or parfait glass, making it look so very elegant.

4   **cups (946 ml) milk**

2   **tablespoons (28 g) Canna-Butter (page 16)**

1   **cup (200 g) granulated sugar**

⅔   **cup (57 g) unsweetened cocoa powder**

¼   **cup (32 g) cornstarch**

¼   **teaspoon salt**

1   **tablespoon vanilla extract**

1. In a medium saucepan over medium-low heat, whisk together the milk and Canna-Butter until the Canna-Butter is melted and the milk is warmed.

2. In a large saucepan over medium heat, combine the sugar, cocoa powder, cornstarch, and salt.

3. Gradually stir the hot milk mixture into the dry ingredients, stirring constantly until smooth.

4. Allow the mixture to simmer gently until thickened, about 7 to 9 minutes. Remove from the heat and stir in the vanilla. Pour into a bowl or individual pudding cups, cover, and chill before serving (if you can stand to wait that long). The pudding will keep, covered, in the refrigerator for up to 4 days.

Yield: Serves 6

CHEF'S NOTE If you want to add a special something, crush a bunch of malted milk balls and add them to the thickened pudding at the end of the cooking time. It's amazing.

RICE PUDDING

A good rice pudding is to comfort desserts what a pot pie is to main courses. The most important thing to remember when cooking this pudding is to be patient. The rice mixture does not thicken much upon cooling, so be sure the rice is soft and the pudding fairly thick before chilling it.

1½ cups (355 ml) water

¾ cup (75 g) basmati rice

Pinch of salt

3 cups (700 ml) half-and-half

1 cup (235 ml) heavy cream or Canna-Cream (page 24)

2 tablespoons (28 g) Canna-Butter (page 16)

½ cup (100 g) granulated sugar

1 tablespoon (15 ml) vanilla extract

1. In a large saucepan, combine the water, basmati rice, and salt and bring to a gentle simmer. Cover and cook for 10 to 12 minutes until the water is absorbed. Check after 8 minutes.

2. Add the half-and-half, cream, Canna-Butter, and sugar and cook over medium heat until the rice is tender, about 35 to 40 minutes, stirring every 10 minutes or so.

3. Remove the pan from the heat and stir in the vanilla. Transfer to a bowl or individual pudding cups, cover, and chill before serving. The pudding will keep, covered, in the refrigerator for up to 4 days.

Yield: Serves 6

CHEF'S NOTE Soak some dried apricots or prunes in bourbon for 30 minutes and then drain and chop and stir into the pudding along with the vanilla. You will have a delightful treat.

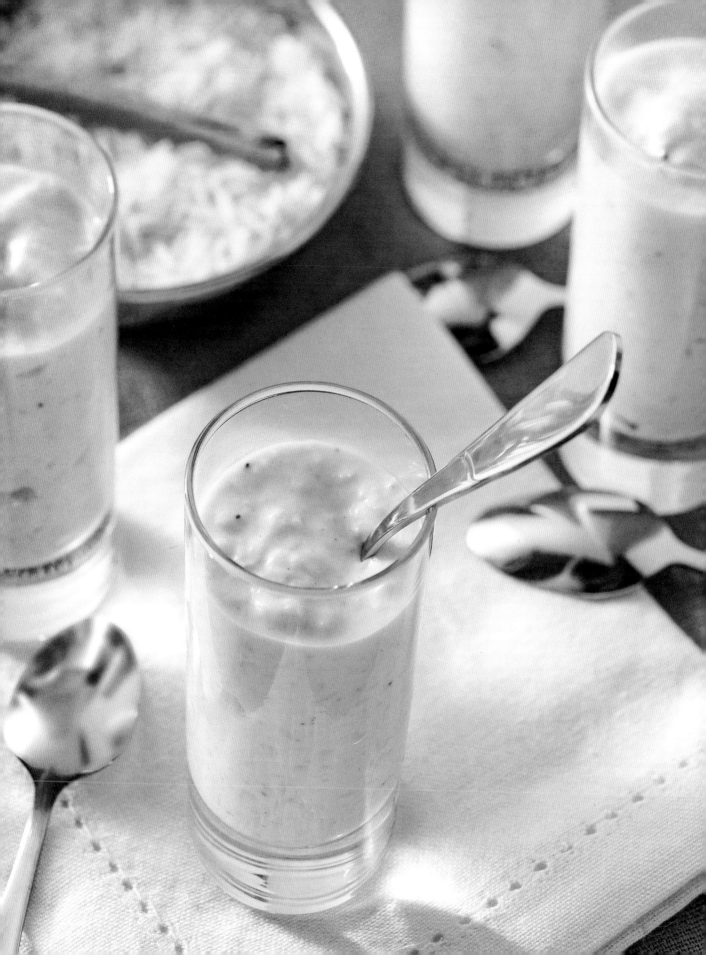

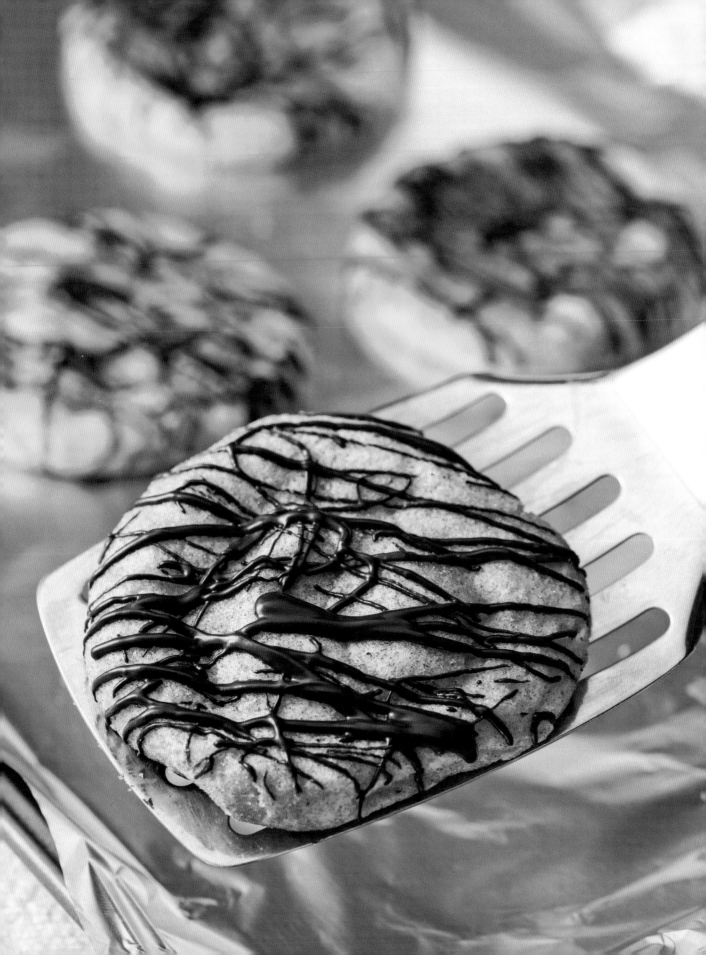

SNICKERDOODLES WITH CHOCOLATE DRIZZLE

With their sugar-cinnamon coating and chewy goodness, snickerdoodles could not possibly get better, it would seem. Well, they just have. With a bit of cannabis and a chocolate drizzle, this cookie may become your new favorite.

COOKIES

2½ cups (313 g) all-purpose flour

2 teaspoons cream of tartar

1 teaspoon baking soda

Pinch of salt

9 tablespoons (126 g) Canna-Butter (page 16), softened

5 tablespoons (70 g) unsalted butter, softened

1½ cups (300 g) granulated sugar, plus ⅓ cup (67 g) for rolling

2 large eggs

1 tablespoon (15 ml) vanilla extract

1½ tablespoons (11 g) ground cinnamon

CHOCOLATE DRIZZLE

1 cup (175 g) chocolate chips

1 tablespoon (14 g) plus 1 teaspoon unsalted butter

1. <u>To make the cookies:</u> Preheat the oven to 340°F (170°C, or gas mark 3) and line baking sheets with parchment paper.

2. In a medium bowl, combine the flour, cream of tartar, baking soda, and salt.

3. In a large bowl using an electric mixer, beat both of the butters and the 1½ cups (300 g) sugar till fluffy. Add the eggs and vanilla and beat till incorporated. Stir in the dry ingredients until there is no flour showing. Chill the dough for 30 minutes.

4. In a small bowl, combine the ⅓ cup (67 g) sugar with the cinnamon. Roll the chilled dough into 36 balls measuring 1½ inches (3.8 cm). Roll the balls in the cinnamon sugar and place 2 inches (5 cm) apart on the prepared baking sheets.

5. Bake for 8 to 10 minutes until set and turning light golden brown. Allow to cool thoroughly on a wire rack.

6. <u>To make the chocolate drizzle:</u> In the top of a double boiler set over simmering water, combine the chocolate chips with the butter. Whisk until melted and smooth.

7. Drizzle the cooled cookies with the chocolate sauce. Allow to set on the rack for at least 30 minutes before serving. The cookies will keep in an airtight container at room temperature for up to 3 weeks.

Yield: Serves 36 (1 cookie per serving)

CHEF'S NOTE Cream of tartar is what sets a snickerdoodle apart from a sugar cookie. It is what's responsible for the slight tanginess of the cookie and its almost pillow-like texture. And a sugar cookie is crunchy, whereas a snickerdoodle is soft. And last but not least, a snickerdoodle has cinnamon!

RED VELVET CUPCAKES

In the old days, the red color in this dessert came from beets. Some folks still use them, but most go for the bottle of food coloring and the knowledge that your fingers will be red for a good portion of the day!

CUPCAKES

2½	cups (280 g) cake flour
3	tablespoons (16 g) unsweetened Dutch-process cocoa powder
½	teaspoon salt
1¼	cups (225 g) granulated sugar
1	cup (235 ml) canola oil
½	cup (120 ml) Canna-Oil (page 18), made with coconut oil
2	large eggs
¼	cup (60 ml) liquid red food coloring
2	teaspoons vanilla extract
1	cup (235 ml) buttermilk
1½	teaspoons baking soda
2	teaspoons white vinegar

FROSTING

1½	sticks (167 g) unsalted butter, softened
4	cups (480 g) confectioner's sugar
2	teaspoons vanilla extract

1. <u>To make the cupcakes:</u> Preheat the oven to 340°F (170°C, or gas mark 3). Spray 2 standard 12-cup muffin pans with cooking spray or line with paper liners.

2. In a medium bowl, combine the cake flour, cocoa powder, and salt.

3. In the bowl of an electric mixer, combine the granulated sugar and both of the oils. Add the eggs, beat until combined, and then add the food coloring and vanilla and beat until blended.

4. Add the dry ingredients to the mixer bowl, alternating them with the buttermilk, and mix until no streaks remain.

5. In a small bowl, combine the baking soda and vinegar. Allow it to foam and then mix it into the batter.

6. Pour the batter into the muffin pans and bake for 18 minutes or until a toothpick stuck in the center of a cupcake comes out clean. Allow to cool on a wire rack.

7. <u>To make the frosting:</u> In the bowl of an electric mixer, beat the butter till fluffy.

8. Slowly add the confectioner's sugar and continue beating. When the sugar is fully incorporated, add the vanilla and mix to incorporate. Frost the cooled cupcakes. The cupcakes will keep in an airtight container at room temperature for up to 3 days or in the refrigerator for up to 5 days. Or freeze the frosted cupcakes for up to 1 month.

Yield: Serves 24 (1 cupcake per serving)

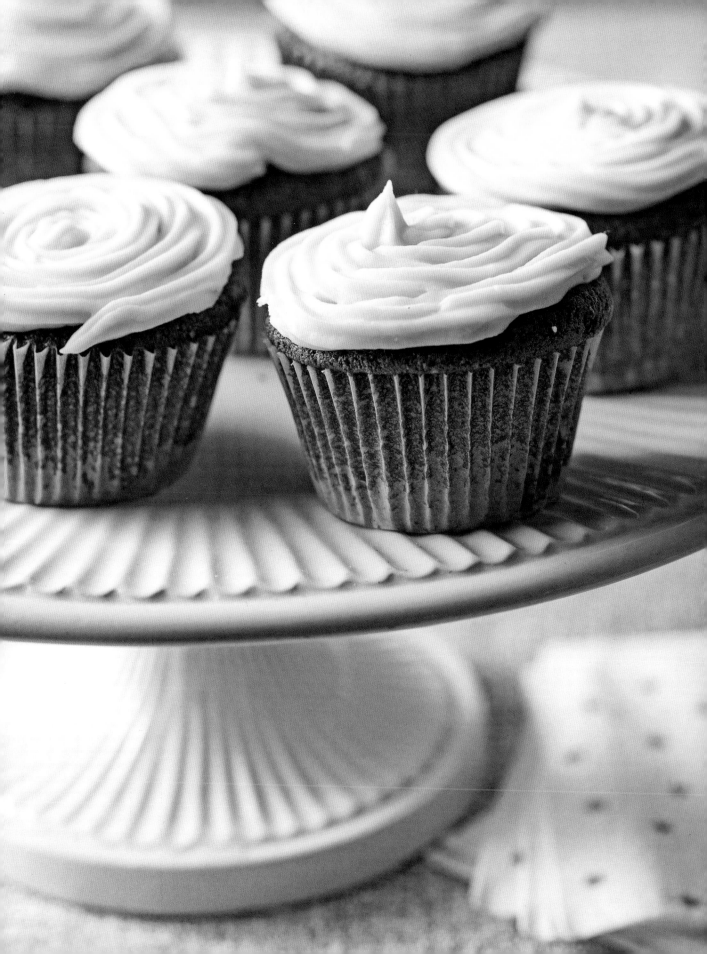

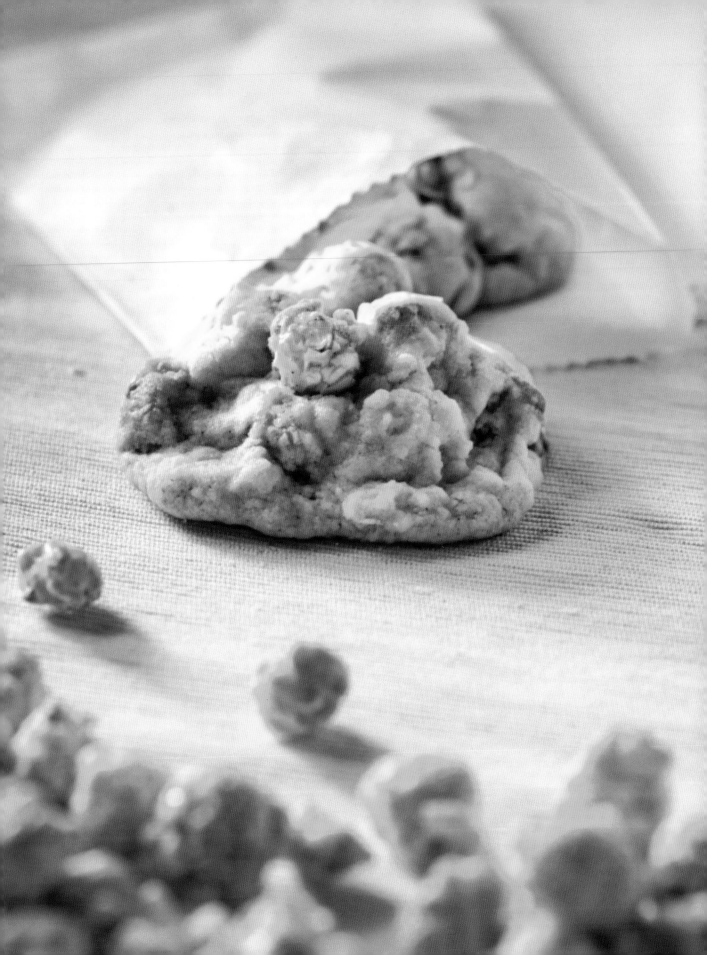

CARAMEL CORN COOKIES

This is one amazing cookie. It is truly munchie magic. You can make the cookies with regular popcorn, without the caramel, but I don't advise it. This version is the way to go.

2¾ cups (344 g) all-purpose flour

1 teaspoon baking soda

½ teaspoon baking powder

Pinch of salt

10 tablespoons (140 g) unsalted butter

6 tablespoons (85 g) Canna-Butter (page 16)

1½ cups (300 g) granulated sugar

1 large egg

1 teaspoon vanilla extract

1½ cups (50 g) caramel corn

1. Preheat the oven to 340°F (170°C, or gas mark 3) and line baking sheets with parchment paper.

2. In a medium bowl, combine the flour, baking soda, baking powder, and salt.

3. In a large bowl using an electric mixer, beat together both of the butters and the sugar till light and fluffy. Add the egg and vanilla and mix to incorporate. Stir in the dry ingredients until no streaks remain. Add the caramel corn and stir gently.

4. Scoop the dough onto the prepared baking sheets in heaping tablespoon (15 g) portions, spacing them 2 inches (5 cm) apart.

5. Bake until light golden brown, about 10 to 12 minutes. Let cool on a wire rack. The cookies will keep in an airtight container at room temperature for up to 2 weeks, though they will begin to lose their crispness after several days.

Yield: Serves 18 (2 cookies per serving)

 CHEF'S NOTE If you are looking for something else to do, drizzle the cookies with some melted chocolate. And maybe sprinkle that melted chocolate with chopped peanuts.

BAKLAVA

Baklava is one of my favorite foods to infuse. Brushing the paper-thin sheets of phyllo dough with Canna-Butter or Canna-Oil is fun. Don't be afraid of phyllo dough; it is incredibly forgiving to work with.

½ cup (112 g) unsalted butter

½ cup (112 g) Canna-Butter (page 16)

1 pound (455 g) mixed unsalted nuts, chopped

1 teaspoon ground cinnamon

1 pound (455 g) phyllo dough, at room temperature

1 cup (235 ml) water

1 cup (200 g) granulated sugar

¾ cup (240 g) honey

1. Preheat the oven to 340°F (170°C, or gas mark 3).

2. In a small saucepan over low heat, melt both of the butters together and pour into a heatproof bowl. Mix the nuts and the cinnamon in another bowl.

3. Place the phyllo dough on your work surface and cover the sheets with a slightly damp kitchen towel.

4. In a 9 x 13-inch (23 x 33 cm) pan, start layering the phyllo sheets. Lay a sheet in the pan and brush gently with the melted Canna-Butter. Continue this way with 12 more sheets, brushing with butter after each layer.

5. Spread the nuts evenly over the brushed sheets.

6. Begin layering more phyllo sheets on top of the nuts, brushing with butter after each new layer. Add another 13 sheets.

7. Using a very sharp knife, carefully cut the dough into 1 x 3-inch (2.5 x 7.5 cm) rectangular or diamond shapes all the way through to the bottom of the pan. Bake for 50 minutes until golden brown.

8. While the baklava is baking, make the sauce. In a small saucepan, combine the water and sugar. Heat over medium heat until the sugar is dissolved, stirring occasionally. Add the honey, lower the heat, and simmer gently for 30 minutes. Remove from the heat.

9. Pour the sauce evenly over the baklava as soon as it comes out of the oven. Allow to cool completely on a wire rack. The baklava will keep in an airtight container at room temperature for up to 5 days.

Yield: Serves 24 (1 piece per serving)

CHEF'S NOTE You can vary the types of nuts according to your own preferences, and though it's not traditional, feel free to add some chocolate chips to the nuts. I once made this dessert with toasted macadamia nuts and white chocolate. It was very rich and very good.

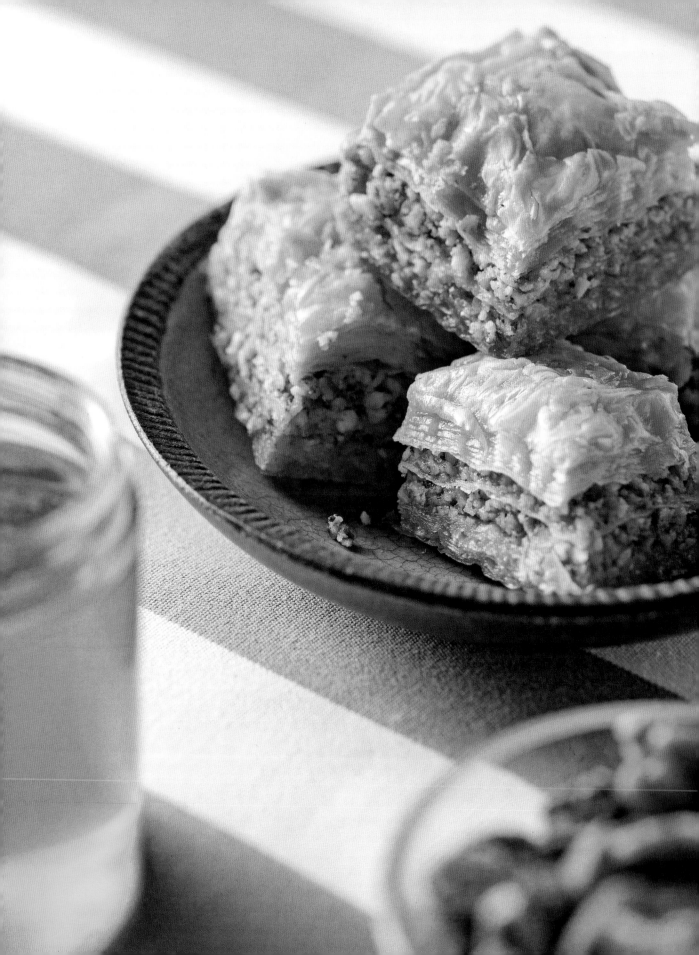

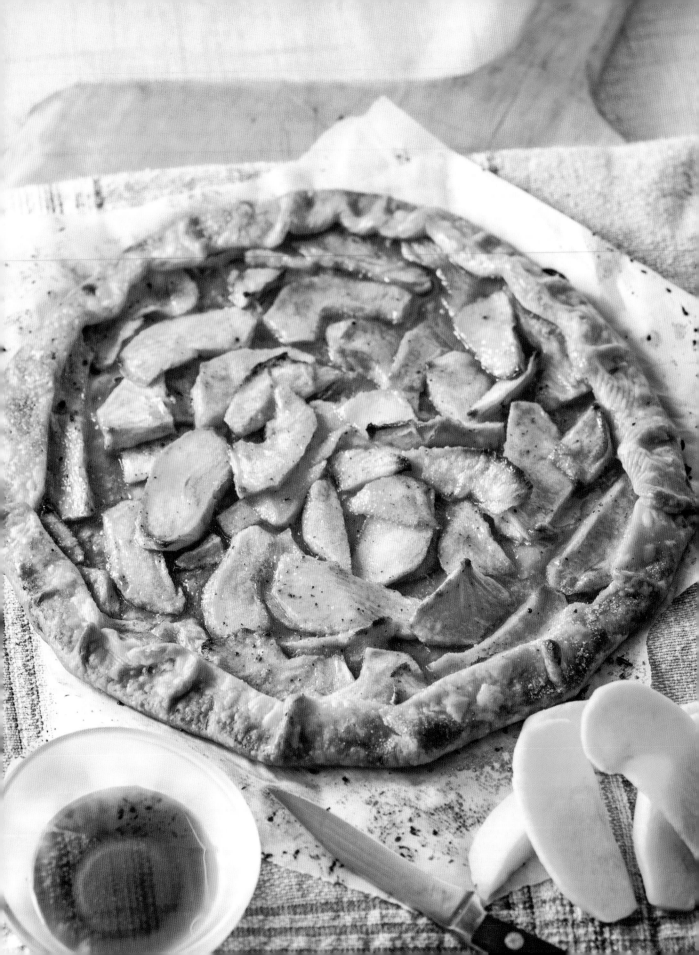

RUSTIC APPLE TART

In the fall, when apples are at their peak, this tart is sublime. If you want to experiment, you could swap the maple syrup for granulated sugar. Feel free to sprinkle a little ground cinnamon or nutmeg on top. And, of course, ice cream is a nice finishing touch.

1   **crust for a 9-inch (23 cm) single-crust pie (store-bought or your favorite recipe)**

3   **tablespoons (42 g) Canna-Butter (page 16), melted**

2   **large apples, peeled, cored, and thinly sliced**

2   **tablespoons (28 ml) maple syrup**

1   **tablespoon (15 ml) fresh lemon juice**

1. Preheat the oven to 340°F (170°C, or gas mark 3).

2. Place the piecrust on your work surface and roll it out to about 11 inches (28 cm). Brush the surface with the melted Canna-Butter and transfer to a baking sheet.

3. In a medium bowl, toss the apples with the maple syrup and lemon juice.

4. Arrange the apples on the crust, leaving about a 1-inch (2.5 cm) space around the edges. Fold the crust edges up gently to create a border. Bake for 25 to 30 minutes until the apples are tender and the crust is golden brown. Let cool on a wire rack for about 10 minutes. Serve warm.

Yield: Serves 9

CHEF'S NOTE   You could also make this tart with frozen puff pastry. A mixture of apples and pears is another way to go for the fruit. And sprinkle some walnuts over the fruit if you are so inclined.

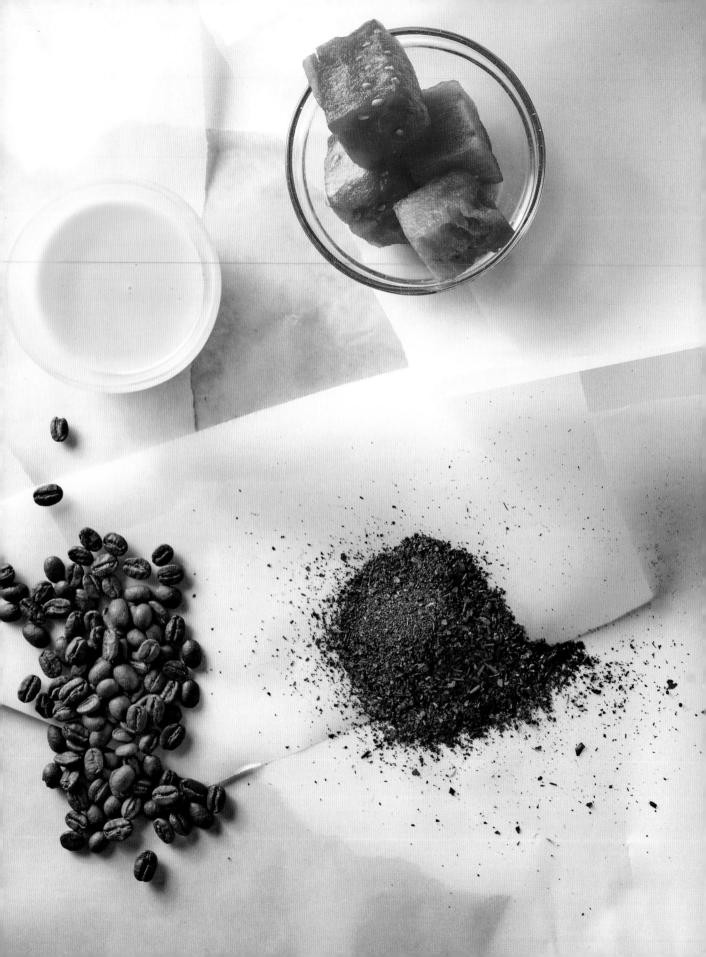

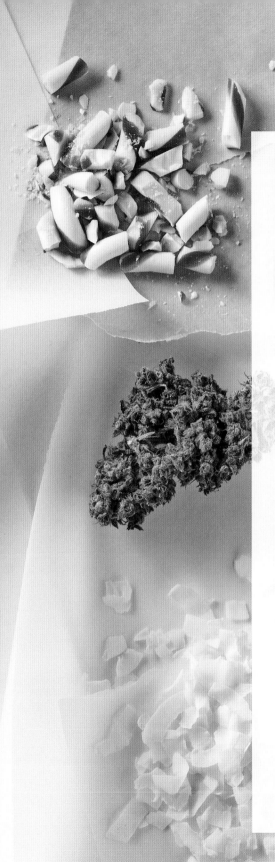

8

BEVERAGES

Beverages can be a little tricky to infuse. If using Canna-Butter or Canna-Oil, the best method is a bit of time in a blender to emulsify the beverage. Simple syrup infused with cannabis is another way to go, and that method infuses and sweetens the beverage at the same time. Simple syrup does not get super potent, so a serving is 1 tablespoon (15 ml), which is 10 mg. In most of the recipes in this chapter, we are infusing the drinks with either Canna-Butter or Canna-Oil, but feel free to experiment by substituting the infused Simple Canna-Syrup on page 22; just remember that a serving is 1 tablespoon (15 ml).

CARAMEL COFFEE

This creamy coffee is great at any time of the day. If you've made your butter with an indica strain, use decaf coffee and you'll sleep like a baby.

2   **cups (475 ml) hot brewed coffee**

1   **cup (235 ml) sweetened condensed milk**

1   **tablespoon (15 g) brown sugar**

2   **teaspoons Canna-Butter (page 16)**

2   **tablespoons (28 g) chopped toffee chocolate bar**

Dusting of unsweetened cocoa powder or ground cinnamon, or both

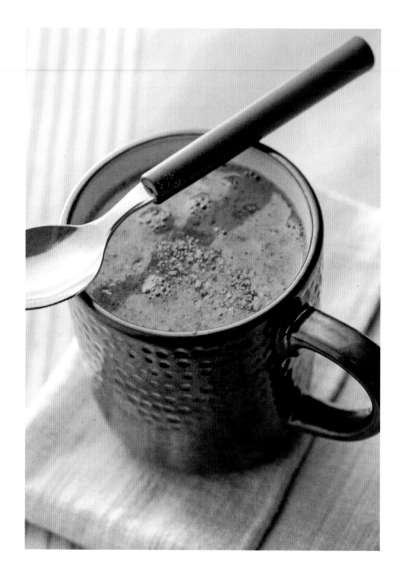

1. In a medium saucepan over medium heat, combine the coffee, condensed milk, brown sugar, and Canna-Butter and cook for 10 to 12 minutes, stirring occasionally.

2. Carefully pour into a blender. Process for 1 to 2 minutes.

3. Divide between 2 heatproof glasses or mugs. Sprinkle with the toffee bits and dust with cocoa, cinnamon, or both!

Yield: Serves 2

CHEF'S NOTE

If you like a little spice, top the coffee with a sprinkling of cayenne pepper or a pure ground chile powder, such as ancho. It's a nice change of pace. This coffee is also yummy served iced.

THAI TEA

This drink is a huge hit whenever I serve it. It's a wonderfully sweet, refreshing drink with a vibrant flavor and beautiful color. I tend to leave out the ice for fear of watering down this cup of gold.

2 **cups (475 ml) water**

½ **cup (48 g) Thai tea leaves or regular black tea leaves**

½ **cup (120 ml) condensed milk**

2 **teaspoons Canna-Butter (page 16)**

1 **teaspoon vanilla extract**

Ice cubes (optional)

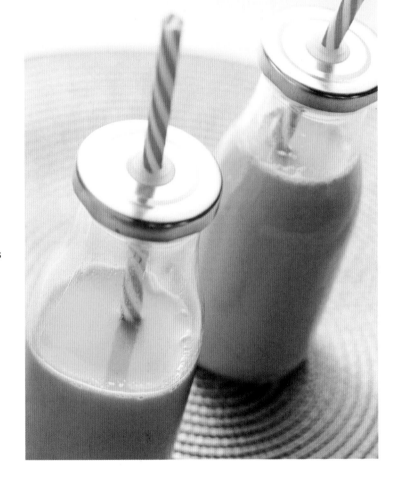

1. Bring the water to a boil in a kettle. Allow to rest for a couple of minutes to bring the temperature down a few degrees and then pour over the tea leaves in a teapot or bowl and let steep for about 4 minutes. Strain.

2. While still hot, add the condensed milk, Canna-Butter, and vanilla. Whisk together to combine thoroughly for at least 1 minute. Place in the fridge to cool.

3. Serve cool, with ice if you like.

Yield: Serves 2

CHEF'S NOTE This drink is also fantastic served warm. If it cools down too much after adding the condensed milk and butter, reheat it over low heat on the stove. For a vegan option, use Canna-Oil made with coconut oil instead of the Canna-Butter and coconut milk instead of the condensed milk.

PEPPERMINT HOT CHOCOLATE

Peppermint and chocolate have been together for years. And they are a lovely couple. Last time I made this, I floated a peppermint patty on top. When that melted, it was heavenly.

3   cups (700 ml) milk

1   cup (235 ml) half-and-half

¼   cup (50 g) granulated sugar

6   ounces (170 g) semisweet chocolate, chopped

4   teaspoons (19 g) Canna-Butter (page 16)

2   drops peppermint extract
    Whipped cream, for serving

4   tablespoons (55 g) crushed peppermint candy, for serving

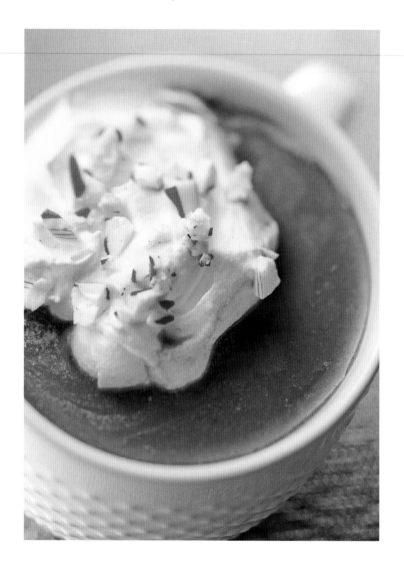

1. In a medium saucepan, heat the milk and half-and-half over medium heat. Stir in the sugar and heat till completely dissolved. Don't let it boil.

2. Add the chocolate and Canna-Butter and stir until melted. Remove from the heat and stir in the extract.

3. Pour into cups, top with the whipped cream, and sprinkle with the crushed candy. Serve immediately.

Yield: Serves 4

CHEF'S NOTE

If peppermint is not your thing, substitute vanilla extract and crushed butterscotch candy for the peppermint extract and peppermint candy.

CHOCOLATE-COCONUT MILK SHAKES

This milk shake is decadent. Chocolate and coconut are a fantastic flavor duo. I can say no more.

2   scoops of dark chocolate ice cream

1   scoop of coconut ice cream

1   cup (235 ml) coconut milk

2   teaspoons Canna-Butter (page 16)

2   tablespoons (28 ml) chocolate syrup

2   tablespoons (11 g) unsweetened shredded coconut, toasted

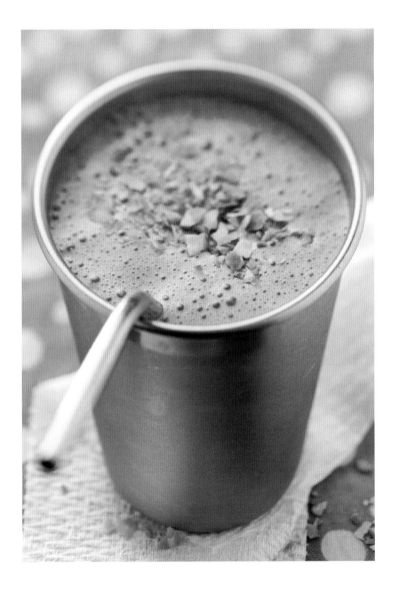

1. In a blender, combine both of the ice creams and the coconut milk. Blend well.

2. Add the Canna-Butter and chocolate syrup and process until you reach the desired consistency.

3. Pour into 2 glasses and sprinkle with the toasted coconut. Serve immediately.

Yield: Serves 2

CHEF'S NOTE To toast coconut, place in a dry nonstick skillet and cook over low heat until golden brown. Remove from the pan right away to prevent it from darkening further and let cool.

WICKED WATERMELON

This drink is sometimes available at Mexican restaurants and markets; it's always tough to decide between this and horchata. You can make this one in less than 5 minutes, so long as you have the simple syrup waiting in the fridge. I would suggest using either Canna-Oil or Simple Canna-Syrup, but not both, unless you have a very high tolerance.

3 **cups (450 g) watermelon chunks**

4 **teaspoons (20 ml) Canna-Oil (page 18), made with coconut oil**

1 **lime, cut into chunks (do not peel)**

¼ **cup (60 ml) simple syrup or Simple Canna-Syrup (page 22)**

Chopped fresh cilantro, for garnish

1. Place all of the ingredients except for the cilantro leaves in the blender. Puree on high speed for about 1 minute.

2. Garnish with the cilantro leaves and serve immediately.

Yield: Serves 4

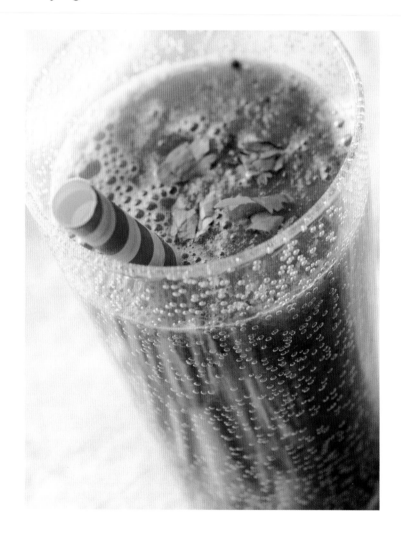

 CHEF'S NOTE If you're feeling adventurous and like spicy foods, add a jalapeño to the blender!

BLUEBERRY LEMONADE

Lemonade from scratch is always a treat. This will keep in the fridge for about 5 days, so feel free to double or triple the recipe.

1 cup (200 g) granulated sugar

1 cup (235 ml) water

2 tablespoons (28 ml) Canna-Oil (page 18), made with coconut oil

1 cup (235 ml) fresh lemon juice

3 cups (700 ml) cold water

1 lemon, thinly sliced

1 cup (145 g) fresh blueberries

1. In a medium saucepan, heat the sugar and water over medium heat till the sugar dissolves. Whisk in the Canna-Oil. Allow to cool.

2. Place the lemon juice and the cooled simple syrup in a large pitcher. Stir to combine. Add the cold water and mix again. Chill until thoroughly cool.

3. Before serving, add the lemon slices and blueberries. Make sure each serving gets a generous amount of blueberries.

Yield: Serves 6

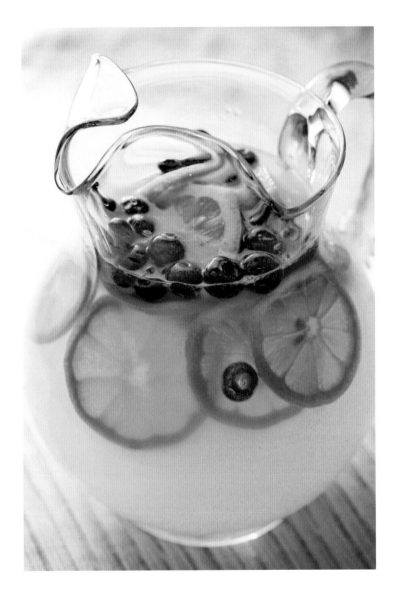

CHEF'S NOTE

If you substitute limes for the lemons, you will have another very refreshing drink.

You can also freeze this mixture in a 9 x 13-inch (23 x 33 cm) baking pan and then run it through your food processor for a terrific granita.

PEANUT BUTTER–ALMOND SMOOTHIES

Made with the right ingredients, a smoothie can take the place of a meal. This one is super-tasty, filling, and good for you—a delicious triple threat.

1   banana, sliced and frozen

8   pitted dates

1½   cups (355 ml) almond milk

¼   cup (60 g) vanilla yogurt

2   tablespoons (32 g) peanut butter

2   tablespoons (28 ml) maple syrup, divided

2   teaspoons Canna-Oil (page 18), made with coconut oil

¼   cup (35 g) chopped roasted unsalted peanuts

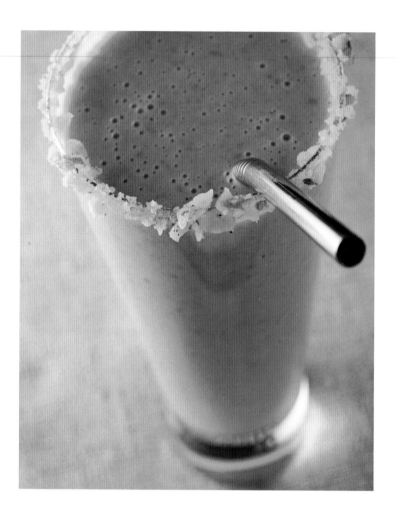

1. In a blender, thoroughly combine the banana, dates, almond milk, yogurt, peanut butter, 1 tablespoon (15 ml) maple syrup, and the Canna-Oil.

2. Place the remaining 1 tablespoon (15 ml) maple syrup on a shallow plate. On another plate, place the peanuts. To rim a glass with peanuts, hold the bottom of the glass, dip the rim in the syrup, and then run it through the peanuts.

3. Pour the smoothie into the prepared glasses and serve.

Yield: Serves 2

SMOOTHIES, SHORT AND SWEET

Smoothies are so versatile—they're a treat any time. For infusing a smoothie, I prefer Canna-Oil made with coconut oil, but Simple Canna-Syrup (page 22) or Canna-Honey (page 28) are also delicious options. Follow these steps for perfect smoothies:

• Place fruit—any kind—in a blender. Use what's in season, or freeze ripe fruit for up to 6 months.

MANGO-COCONUT SMOOTHIES

Besides being incredibly refreshing, this smoothie has a wonderful tropical taste. When mangos are perfectly ripe, they're simply amazing. If you want to go with just mangos, substitute the pineapple with a second mango.

1	**ripe mango, peeled, pitted, and cut into chunks**
1	**cup (165 g) pineapple chunks**
1	**small orange, cut into chunks (do not peel)**
1	**cup (235 ml) coconut milk or coconut water**
2	**tablespoons (28 ml) fresh lime juice**
2	**tablespoons (40 g) honey**
2	**teaspoons Canna-Oil (page 18), made with coconut oil**

Place all of the ingredients in a blender. Pulse to start and then blend on high until smooth. Serve immediately.

Yield: Serves 2

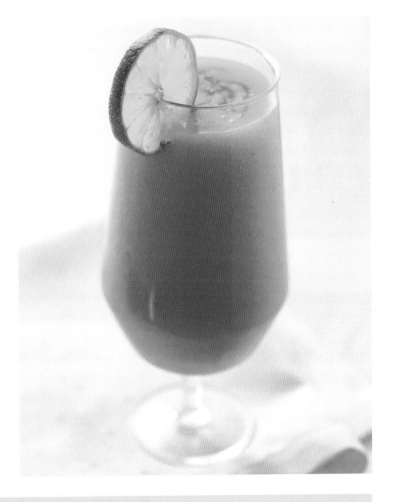

- Add your liquid of choice: fruit juice, various dairy or plant-based milks—even water will work. Add yogurt for a hint of tartness, creaminess, and the health benefits it provides.
- At this point, you can add a variety of flavorings, such as peanut butter, chia seeds or flaxseeds, protein powder, sweeteners, wheat germ, ground cinnamon, or ginger.

- If you want a thick smoothie, add ice—the more, the frothier. If you're using frozen fruit, you may not need it, but for a super-thick treat, add about 1 cup (225 g).

VIRGIN MOJITOS

For many years, I was the food editor of a parenting magazine. Fun ice cubes were often on my summer menus. But they're not just for kids, so I decided to make some pretty ones for this very grown-up drink. The instructions in the note call for using water, but it's also great to use limeade instead. (And that way, your mojito doesn't get watered down.) I suggest making these with either Canna-Oil or Simple Canna-Syrup, but not necessarily both.

3   limes, thinly sliced

Bunch of fresh mint

1   can (6 ounces, or 175 ml) limeade concentrate

¼   cup (60 ml) simple syrup or Simple Canna-Syrup (page 22)

2   cups (475 ml) cold water

4   teaspoons (20 ml) Canna-Oil (page 18), made with coconut oil

Ice cubes, for serving

In a medium pitcher, combine the limes, mint, simple syrup, limeade concentrate, water, and Canna-Oil. Stir well. Serve over ice.

Yield: Serves 4

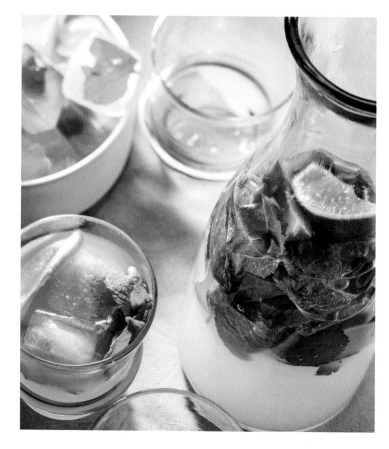

CHEF'S NOTE

I like to serve these mojitos with fun ice cubes. Place your ice cube trays on your work surface. Place raspberries and mint leaves in the compartments of an ice cube tray. Pour water over the berries and mint to fill the compartments halfway and press the berries and mint down into the water. Freeze the tray for 20 minutes and then fill the compartments to the top with water and freeze until set.

VIRGIN SANGRIA

Alcohol has never been my thing—no beer, no wine. I do love a fruity sangria or a tart mojito, but I think that has nothing to do with the alcohol and is more about just the flavors. So being able to infuse these drinks that I enjoy with cannabis has been a terrific revelation. It's life-changing, in fact.

1   cup (150 g) cubed watermelon

⅔   cup (83 g) fresh raspberries

⅔   cup (113 g) sliced fresh strawberries

1   can (6 fluid ounces, or 175 ml) frozen orange juice concentrate

1   cup (235 ml) Simple Canna-Syrup (page 22)

4   cups (946 ml) water

1   cup (235 ml) club soda
    Ice cubes, for serving

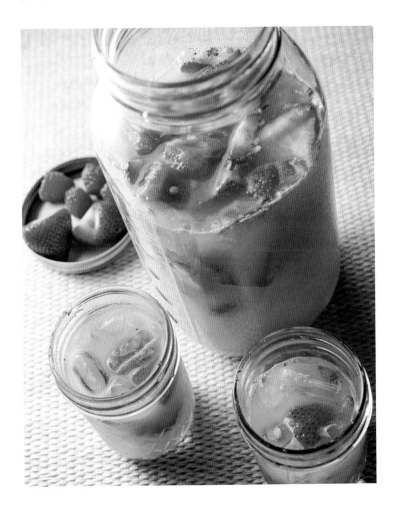

1. In a large pitcher, combine the watermelon, raspberries, strawberries, orange juice concentrate, Simple Canna-Syrup, and water. Mix and chill for 1 hour.

2. When ready to serve, add the club soda and ice cubes.

Yield: Serves 4 to 6

ACKNOWLEDGMENTS

Thank you to Joy, who was actually appropriately named, and is a wise and wonderful editor and just a pleasure to do business with.

Thanks to every lovely person—and there have been many—in this crazy canna-business, including: Oregon's finest, Megan, Selena, and Andrea; Tyler Hurst, for being hugely helpful with his impressive knowledge about all things cannabis and his way with words; Keisha; Alex; my peanut butter friends; Zim from Victory Gardens—a huge thanks; Kip, from Kings of Canna—awesome always; Oscar and his amazing grow store, Portland Organics—you rock; Alex from Chem History— you're the best; and the folks from HiFi Farms—loving our collaborations.

To my non-cannabis-related friends, thank you for your support and enthusiasm. I am fortunate to have such wonderful people around me. And it's not because of the cannabis!

My family has been incredibly supportive during my journey into the fascinating and fun world of cannabis. Thanks to Bruce, who takes the most beautiful photos; Mary, who makes going to work so much fun; and Nick and Olivia, my smart, funny, and helpful adult kids. Thank you all for being there. Or here.

ABOUT THE AUTHOR

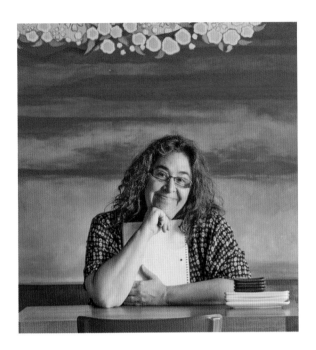

Laurie Wolf is a trained chef who is enjoying the legalization of marijuana in Oregon and thinks that cannabis is a very impressive herb. Laurie attended the Culinary Institute of America after New York University and now lives in Portland, Oregon. She has written two books about the food in Portland and one about the Seattle food scene, as well as several craft books, including *The Lonely Sock Puppet*. With her business partner, Mary Wolf, Laurie co-owns Laurie & MaryJane, an award-winning edibles company. Check out their website, www.laurieandmaryjane.com. Don't fear the edible!

ABOUT THE PHOTOGRAPHER

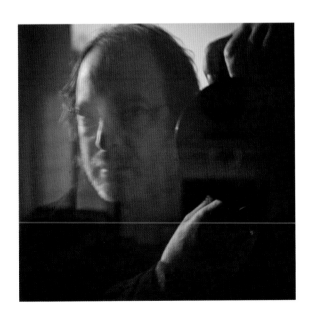

Bruce Wolf is an award-winning photographer whose photos make my food look pretty spectacular. "We like the same music, we like the same bands, we like the same clothes!" (Inside joke.)

INDEX